Muffin Mornings

Nourishing Recipes for
Your Best Life
by
Dominique Battles

P | Pandion Press |

Cover art by Grace Mitchell
Layout by Grace Mitchell
Photographs by Grace Mitchell

ISBN: 978-0-9984262-3-5

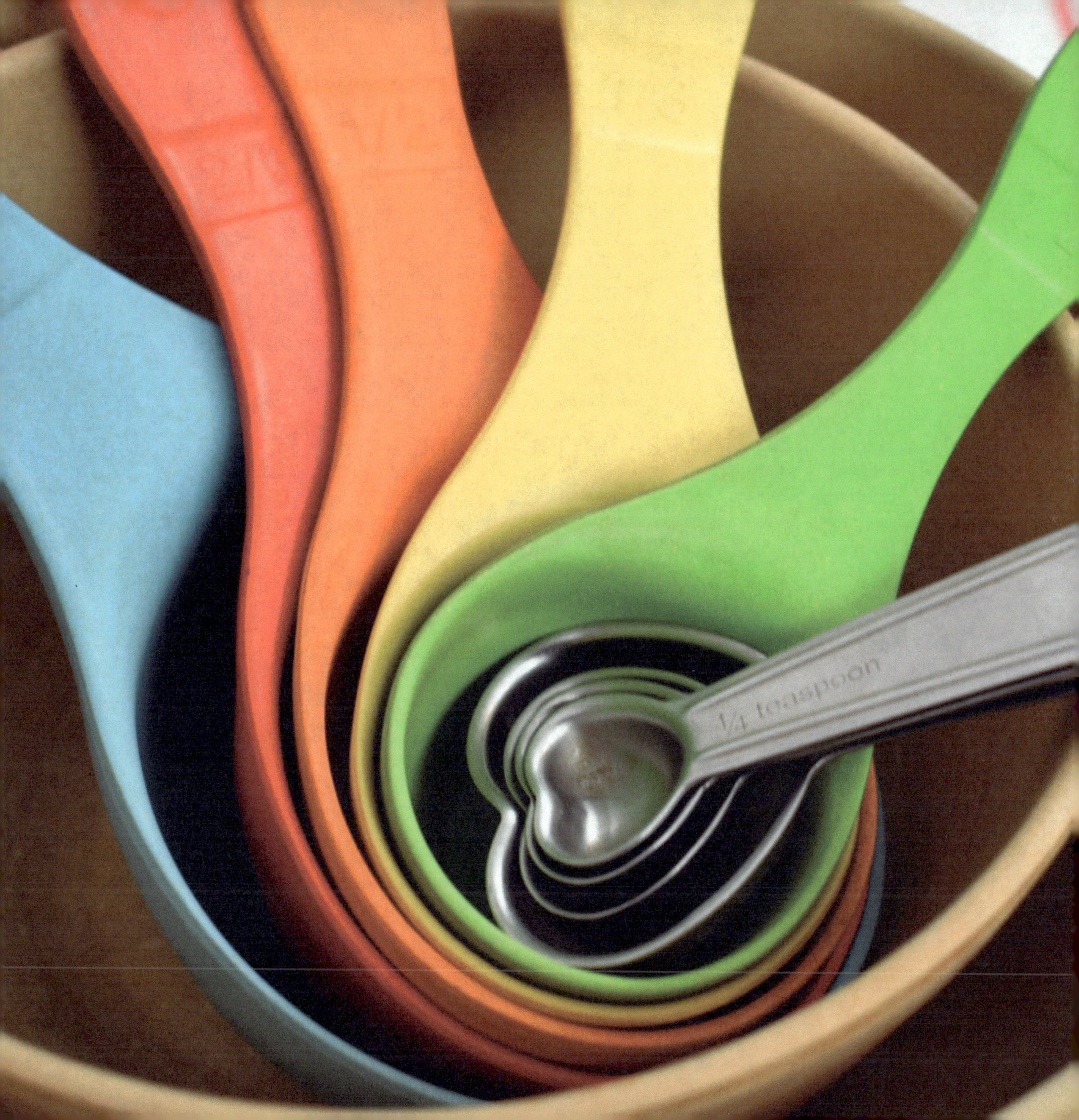
1/4 teaspoon

For my family and their loving enthusiam for my baking endeavors.

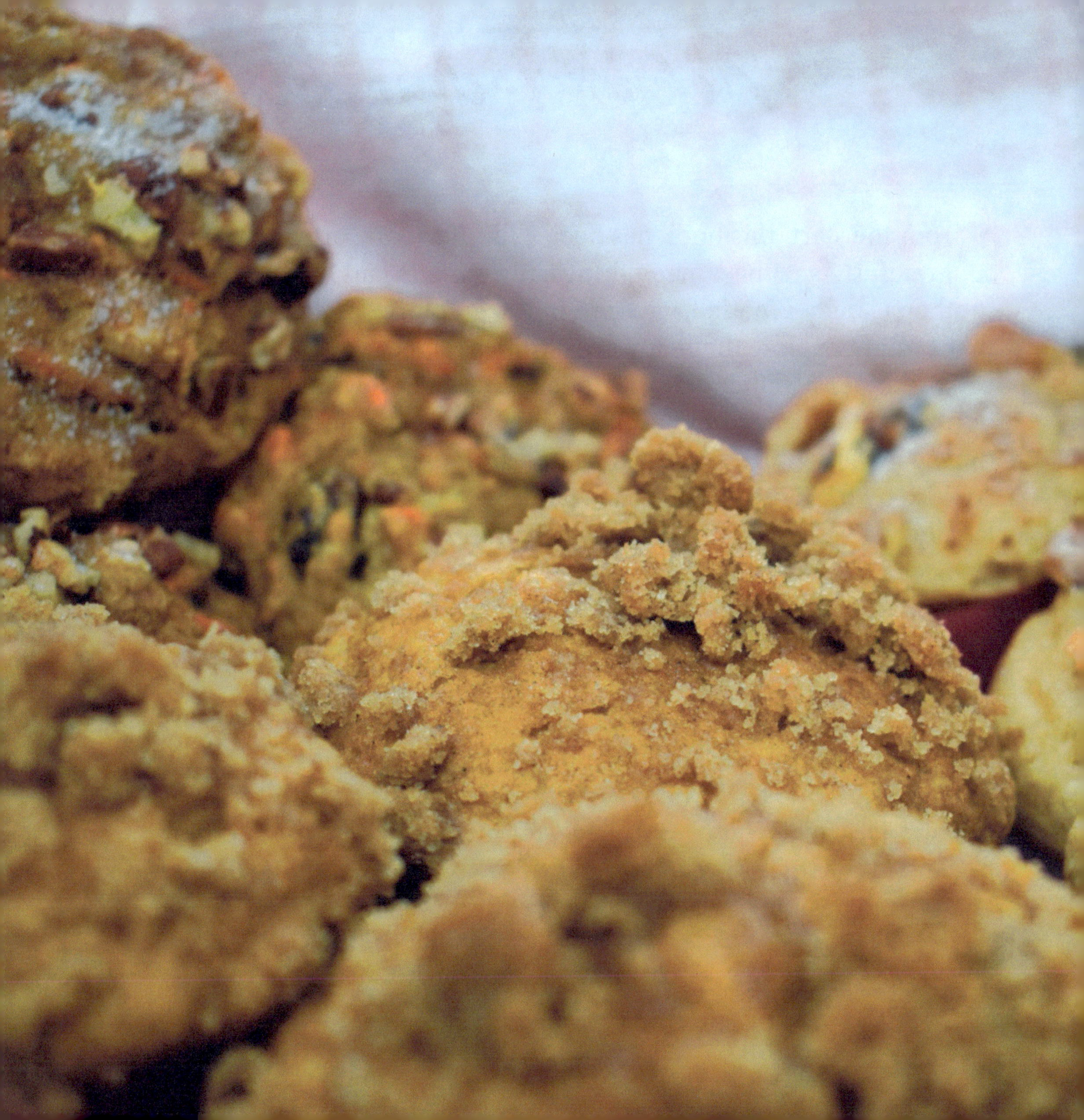

Acknowledgments

From the start, this book has been a family affair for which I am deeply grateful. As with so many things, my parents laid the foundations. My mother, Camay Woodall, gave me full reign of the kitchen early on, so that I might explore the many possibilities it held, and bought me my first cookbooks. My father, Jerry Woodall, quite unknowingly, inspired this book by teaching me how to enrich life through baking when, years ago, during power outages at our Kansas farmhouse, he baked us chocolate chip cookies by the light of a kerosene lamp. My husband, Paul Battles, not only loyally taste-tested each of the recipes in this book over many years, but also coached me through the complex process of book production. My son, Perry Battles, is living proof that homemade muffins build strong human beings, and applied his knowledge of healthy nutrition by providing the nutritional facts for each recipe.

My Hanover family has provided the essential tools for realizing the abiding dream of this book. My deep gratitude goes to Rick Lostutter, Director of Art and Design at Hanover College, for facilitating the production of this book, and to Grace Mitchell for her tireless dedication in its illustration, layout, and design.

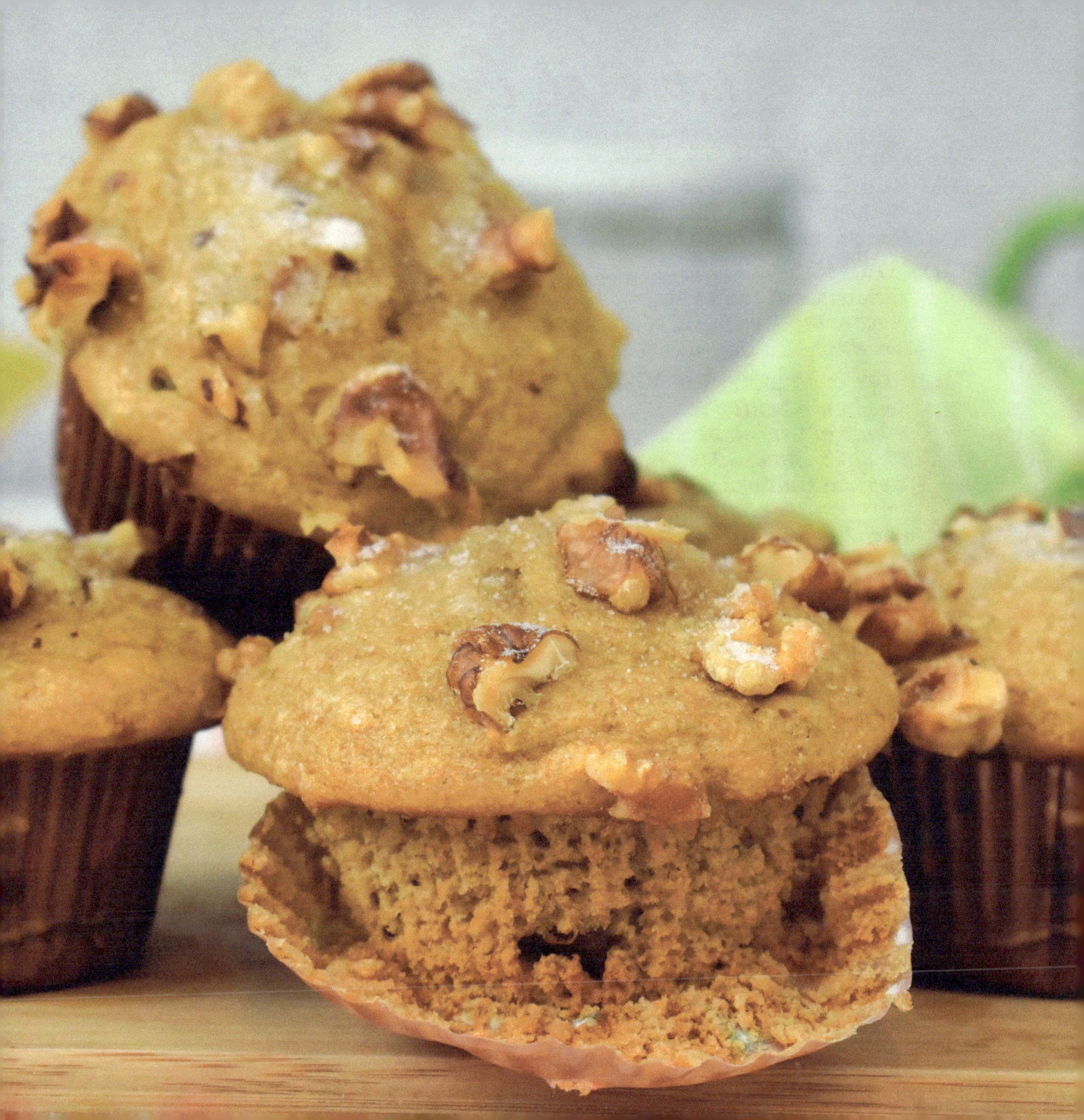

Table of Contents

Introduction

"Our simplest pleasures are rarely simple."
J.B. Priestley

I titled this book the way I did because I came to realize some years ago that the way you spend the first moments of the day shapes all the remaining moments of the day. Whether you're facing a busy day full of active kids and/or absorbing professional commitments, gathering for a festive family brunch, or whether you have the luxury to sit in a quiet chair watching the first birds at the feeder, a healthy, homemade muffin can help bring forth your best life, today.

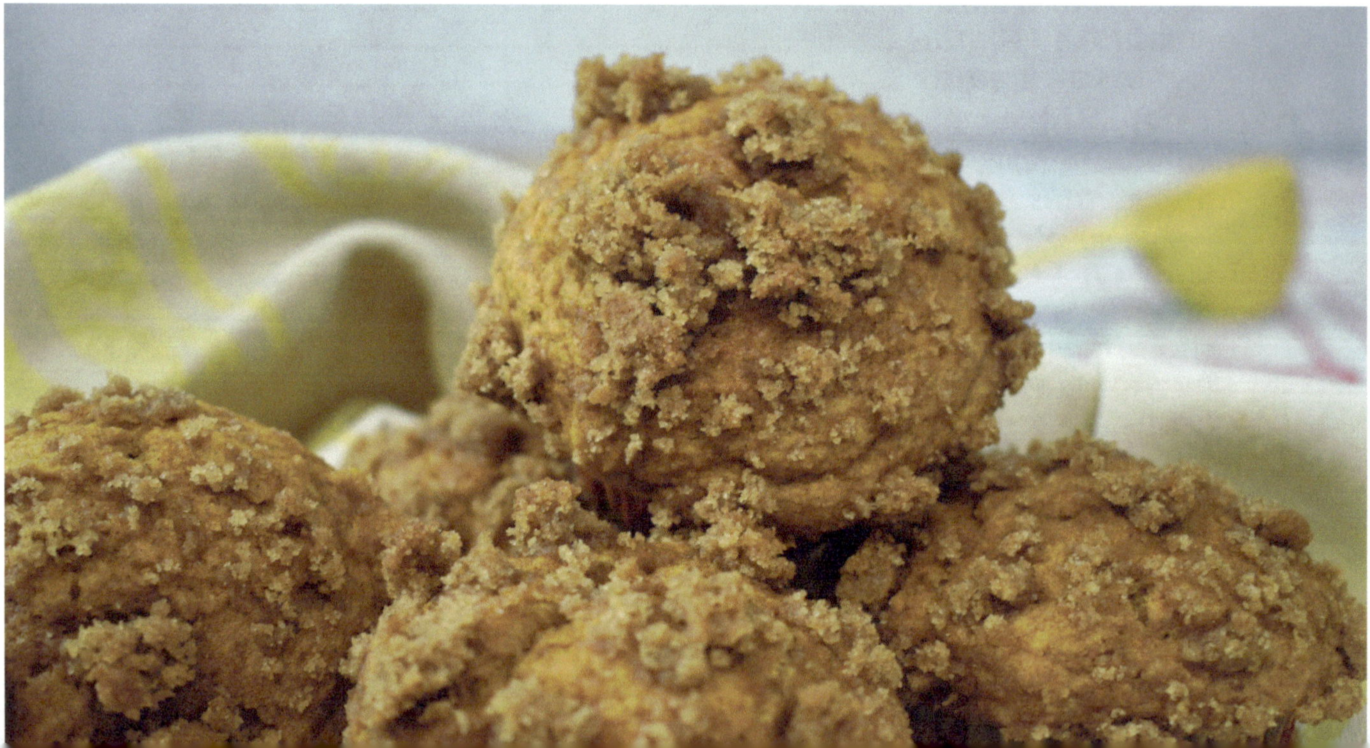

My Journey to the Muffin Top

I never set out to create a muffin book. Rather, I set out to fashion a life worth living, and muffins have been a pillar of that endeavor right from the start.

I began collecting and developing muffin recipes as a teenager in the days before email, or cell phones, or any of our current means of scouting and sharing recipes. With no cookbooks yet to my name, I started with those little box mixes commonly sold in grocery stores, baking up bran and corn muffins after school, and feeling very grown up in doing so. I transitioned from mixes to real baking, from scratch, with the Good Housekeeping Cookbook, a Christmas present from my mom, making each variation of its basic muffin recipe, and then some. So began my life-long fascination with muffins. From college to career, I kept baking, turning each tiny apartment into home with cinnamon, vanilla, and toasted nuts. Once I moved into marriage and motherhood, I began adapting my growing recipe collection in light of nutrition science, incorporating as much whole grain, natural sweeteners, and organic fruit and nuts as good taste would allow, never compromising on sheer deliciousness.

The present volume is but the fanciest version of a muffin cookbook that has been in the making for forty years. Like all beginnings, the start of the collection was humble, with ideas, ingredients, and baking tools imperceptibly slipped in between more important things in life. Over the years, these muffin recipes have grown and graduated from anonymous scribblings on 3"x5" index cards, tucked into the pages of various "official" cookbooks on my kitchen shelf, to an "authored" booklet printed in standard black and white font and stapled by a skilled copy machine, to a three-ring binder of recipes printed on colored paper in a large, playful font and illustrated with copyright-free retro clip-art. However, at the urgings of family and friends who always eagerly anticipate "the muffin this week," I decided the time had come to usher these recipes from my kitchen to yours, confident that they will enrich your life as they have mine, in more ways than one.

The good news for you about this slow, unintentional journey is that each of these recipes has undergone countless revisions over countless years, always with an eye to better nutrition and taste, and only those recipes with superior flavor and texture, and consistent performance, made it in. My sincerest wishes for your happy baking.

How Muffins Improve Life

Versatility

Muffins make a wonderful, hot breakfast that fills the morning with good smells. They are also a perfect tea/coffee time treat, or a snack for the road that makes the world feel friendlier.

Nutrition

Standard muffins, both store-bought and homemade, tend to consist primarily of refined flour and staggering quantities of refined sugar, not to mention questionable fats. All the muffin recipes in this book start with whole meal flour, seeds, nuts, dried or fresh fruit, and healthy fats, supporting body as well as soul. For more nutritional strategies, see below.

Convenience

All of the recipes in this book can be prepared in one bowl in about 15 minutes or less, and baked in less than 20 minutes. Your timing improves with practice.

Cheap Delight

Not many things in life can bring deep pleasure to a gathering of hungry souls for under five dollars, but muffins are one of them. If you want to take your muffin baking experience to the next level, scout out muffin/cupcake papers for every season or holiday (or every mood). How often can you get so much delight for so little money?

Techniques of Muffin Magic

Some basic moves will help to ensure great muffins every time:

Mixing dry and wet ingredients just to combine. In each recipe, I remind bakers to "avoid overmixing," and while I hesitated to repeat this phrase so often, it truly is a make-or-break affair in that overmixing exhausts the rising action of the leavening agent (baking powder or baking soda), preventing your muffins from rising properly. I ruined many a decent muffin early on before I realized what I was doing wrong, so trust me on this one.

Not overbaking. This is another recurring instruction throughout this book. Just like cookies, which are chewiest when slightly underbaked, muffins are moistest when slightly underbaked. If the recipe indicates "bake for 16-18 minutes," I recommend checking them at 16 minutes, and then checking every 60-90 seconds after that, taking them out when the tops still feel a bit doughy. Baking them beyond that point makes them food for squirrels.

Sprinkling rather than folding in the nuts: Most muffin recipes have you fold the chopped nuts into the batter before baking. If, however, you sprinkle the nuts over the batter just before putting them in the oven, the nuts get "roasted" during baking, bringing out their full flavor and aroma. (I discovered this by accident one morning). This technique also enables you to customize your muffins with different nuts (or none, at all) for different palates. My husband adores hazelnuts, and I'm pecans all the way, while my son often wants plain tops. This technique accommodates everyone.

Redeeming those weekday mornings. If you want hot muffins on a busy weekday morning while still getting your beauty rest, mix the dry ingredients together in a bowl with a snap-on lid the night before. The next morning, simply add the wet ingredients while the oven pre-heats. The muffins can be baking while you shower and get the coffee going. Life becomes more civilized and joyous.

Tools of the Trade

Here are the basic tools you will need to start baking those yummy muffins:

- A set of mixing bowls.
- Mixing bowls with snap-on lids (only if you like to pre-mix dry ingredients the night before to save time in the morning).
- A set of measuring cups.
- A set of measuring spoons.
- A wooden spoon that feels great in your hand.
- A 12-16 cup muffin pan.
- Liners for the muffin cups.

While you can certainly do without muffin liners by greasing your muffin pan, the liners make clean-up so much easier. Paper liners work well, and are available in lovely colors and prints, but some of the muffin sticks to them, leaving less for you. Silicon muffin liners leave the muffin fully intact, and have the advantage of being reusable and easy to clean. On the other hand, shopping for pretty paper liners is one of life's endearing pleasures. Something to consider as you prepare to bake.

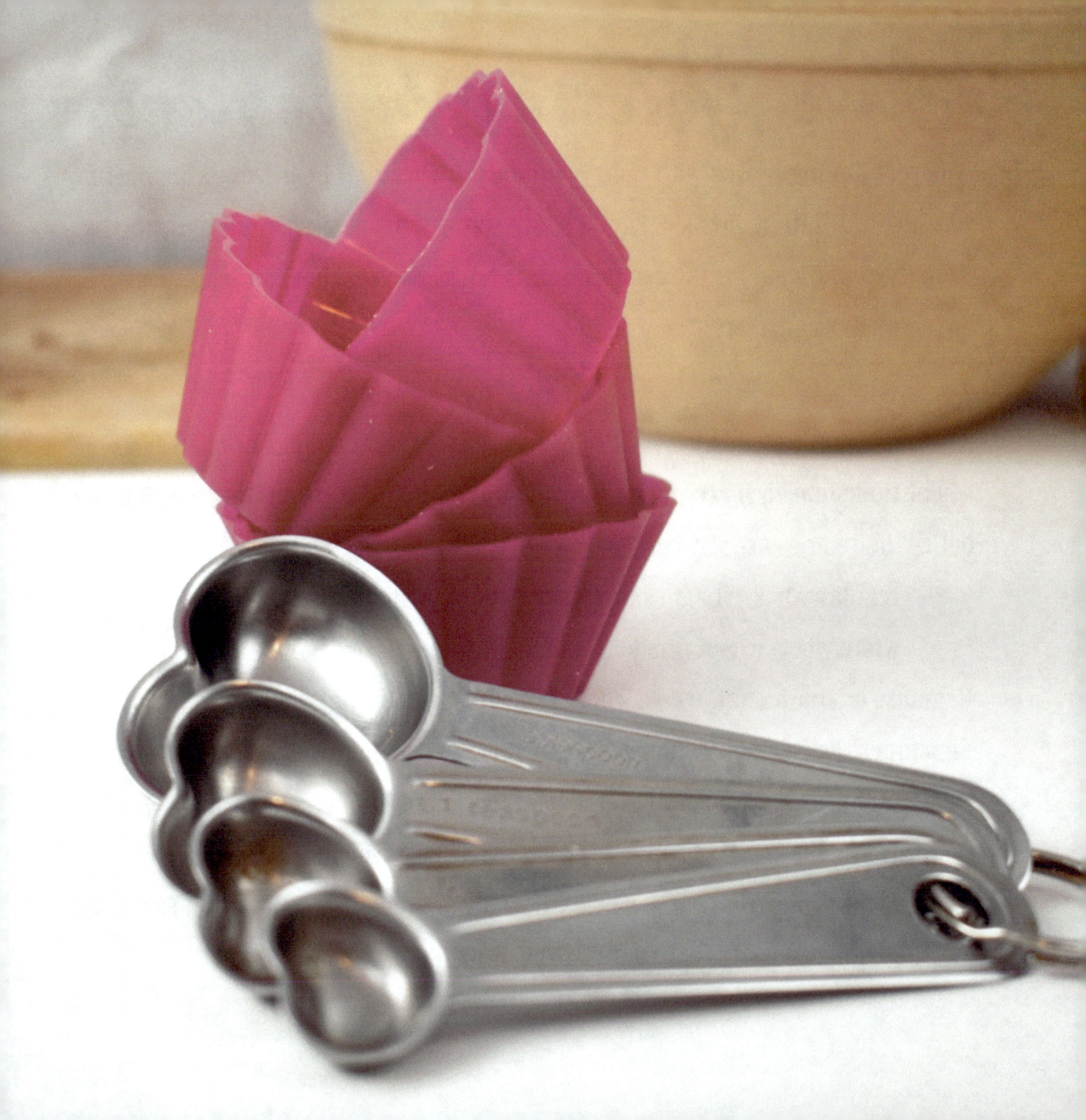

Some Notes on Ingredients

All great baking begins with quality ingredients. And all healthy baking begins with healthful ingredients. Below, I share some of my choices in ingredients that form the foundation for the recipes in this book, choices that can inspire your own growth as a baker.

Flour

As I am committed to good health as well as good taste, I incorporate whole wheat flour into each recipe, for muffins high in fiber and full in flavor. You will notice the recipes usually call for two types of whole wheat flour:

- regular whole wheat flour (made from red wheat), and
- white whole wheat (made from hard white wheat).

Regular, or traditional, whole wheat flour has a deep, nutty flavor, but can sometimes taste gritty. White whole wheat flour has a milder flavor, making it ideal for baking. I have found that a combination of both types of whole wheat flour affords the depth of flavor from regular whole wheat and the lightness of texture and flavor from white whole wheat. Combined with some white flour, you won't even notice you're eating a healthy muffin!

Over the years, I have experimented with common grocery store flours, and commercially available specialty flours, organic and non-organic, and the offerings grow each year. More recently, I have become a devotee of baking flours available in bulk at our little local Mennonite grocery store which brighten the flavor of my biscuits, cookies, cakes, and of course muffins. As you work with the recipes in this book, play around with different brands of flour – they're not all alike.

Oils

For optimally moist muffins, I tend to bake with oil, and less often with butter. For those of us aiming for healthful food, the "oil wars" of recent years over healthy vs. unhealthy fats seem to leave us with fewer and fewer reliable options. The one oil that has remained unscathed in the fray is olive oil, as it delivers unqualified health benefits which survive even cooking at high temperatures. It also has the best record for the allergically sensitive, unlike many nut oils. Fortunately, major olive oil brands now offer an "extra light," virtually flavorless version of the oil perfect for baking that does not overwhelm the lighter flavors of baked goods. So, the "oil" in these recipes means extra-light olive oil. Again, approach your muffin baking with an open mind, and try substituting other healthy oils from various nuts, seeds, and avocado depending on your palate.

Dairy

Most of the recipes in this book call for dairy in the form of milk, buttermilk, or sour cream, in which case I have relied on low-fat options: 2% milk, low-fat buttermilk, or low-fat sour cream. While you can certainly substitute full-fat alternatives, the nutritional information provided for each muffin is calculated for low-fat dairy.

Sweeteners

While lots of muffin recipes out there call for whole grain flours, fresh or dried fruit, and nuts, the high quantities of refined sugar, so often called for in the recipe, compromise any health benefits we might be getting from the good stuff. To better support gut health, these recipes are sweetened with honey, very occasionally supplemented with small amounts of brown sugar or molasses. Honey digests more slowly than refined sugar, helping to avoid the blood sugar spike and insulin response associated with sugar. Honey also contains trace vitamins and minerals not found in sugar. The muffin top is the one domain I researve for a sprinkling of white sugar, or cinnamon sugar, and that little bit is enough. You'll see.

Flavorings

Most of these muffin recipes call for vanilla extract. Some years ago, I began making my own, and I find it is well worth the effort, and really not that hard to do. Purchase five or six tall vanilla beans (the glossiest ones are the freshest), score them lengthwise with a paring knife, pry them open like a book, plunk them into a tall glass jar with a stopper lid, fill the jar with vodka, and place it in a cupboard for three months. When it is almost time, add a couple of teaspoons of sugar to the jar and shake well. More recently, a friend introduced me to specialty vanilla-orange extract, lovely in certain of these muffins. In the absence of this rarer flavoring, you can simply add some orange zest to the recipe along with the vanilla.

As for almond extract, I tread lightly. The recipes that call for it indicate only a drop, and no more than ¼ teaspoon. Any more than that, and you'll taste only almond.

Applesauce

Most of the muffin recipes in this book get some of their moistness and nutrition from applesauce. I always recommend unsweetened, plain (rather than chunky), preferably organic applesauce. Other recipes get their moistness and texture from pumpkin, carrots, squash, or other puréed fruit, but applesauce is the most common one, so I do recommend always having it on hand.

Chocolate

Many life situations simply require chocolate, and you will find a number of muffin recipes in this book to aide you. I recommend organic, semi-sweet chocolate chips, and – for maximum distribution – mini chips over large ones, but you make the call.

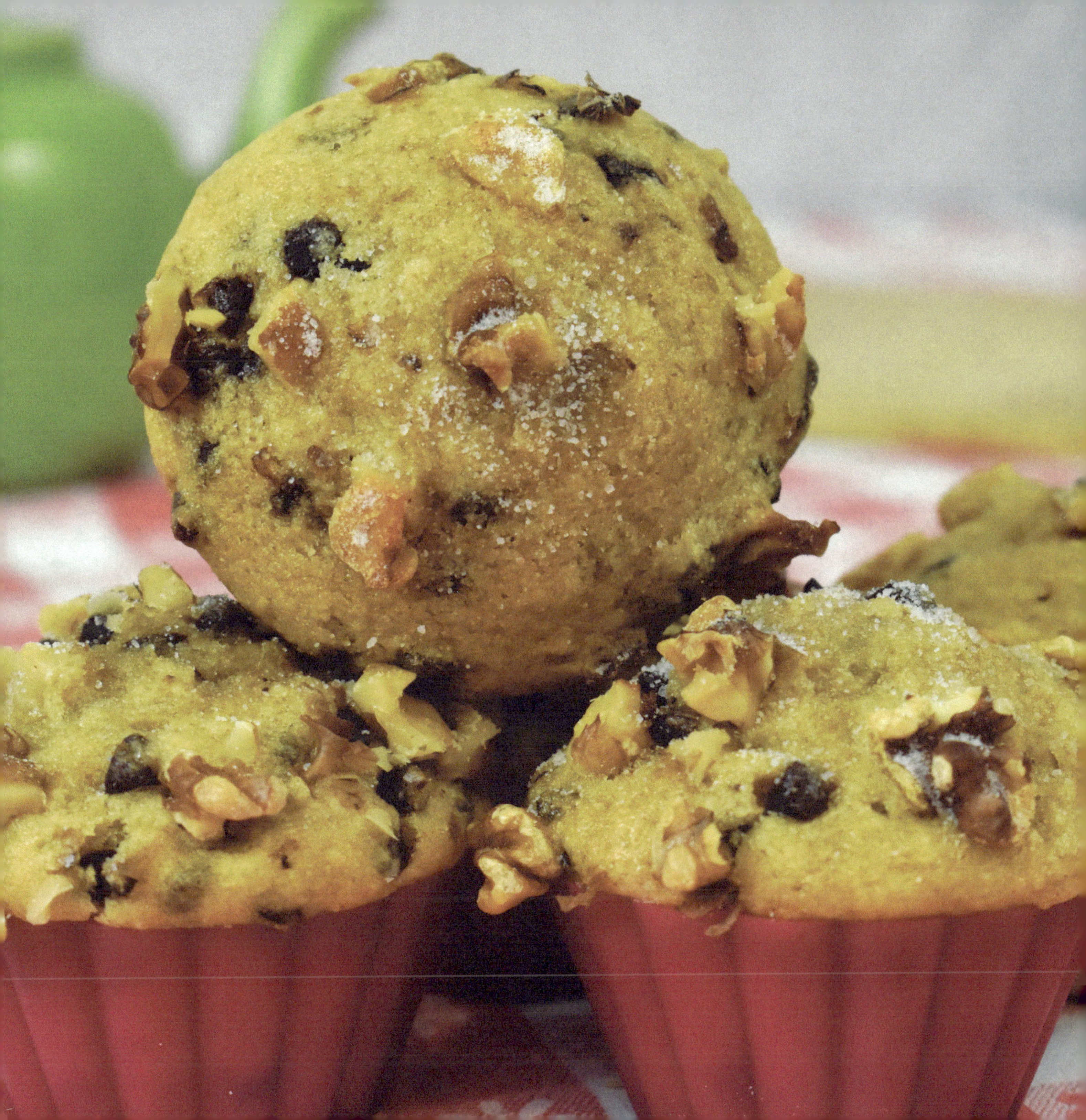

Chapter 1

Veggies for Vitality

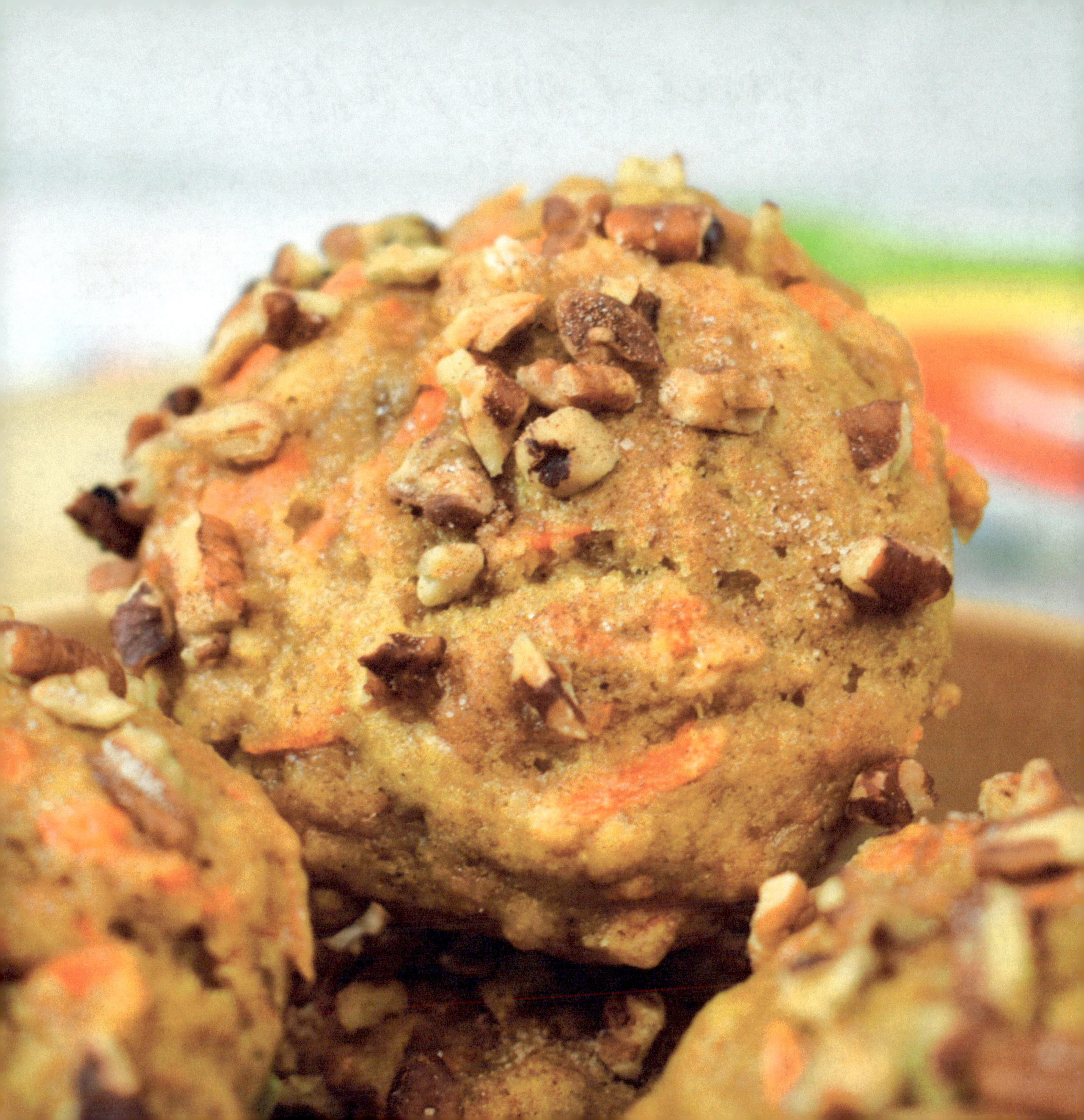

Sweet Corn Muffins

1 cup white whole wheat flour
¼ cup white flour
¾ cup yellow cornmeal
⅛ teaspoon salt
⅓ cup honey
1 Tablespoon baking powder
½ cup milk
½ cup applesauce
2 eggs
2 Tablespoons oil
1 teaspoon vanilla

Sweeter and moister than traditional corn bread.

1. Preheat oven to 350 degrees F.
2. In a medium bowl, mix together the dry ingredients.
3. Make a well in the center and add the wet ingredients.
4. Stir just to combine (avoid overmixing).
5. Spoon batter into muffin cups.
6. Bake for 15-20 minutes. (Best if a bit underbaked.)
7. Note: These muffins are best on the first day.
   Makes 12 muffins

Per Muffin

Calories: 144
Fat: 4g
Cholesterol: 32mg
Sodium: 165mg

Potassium: 39mg
Carbs: 25g
Fiber: 2g
Sugars: 9g
Protein: 4g

Vitamin A: 17%
Vitamin C: 8%
Calcium: 86%
Iron: 4%

Pumpkin-Date Muffins

The rum and dates in these makes a special and nutritious variation on the basic pumpkin muffin.

- 1 cup white whole wheat flour
- 1 cup white flour
- 2 Tablespoons brown sugar
- 2 teaspoons baking powder
- ½ teaspoon baking soda
- 1 ¼ teaspoons cinnamon
- ¼ teaspoon cloves
- ¼ teaspoon ginger
- ⅛ teaspoon salt
- ½ cup honey
- ½ cup chopped dates
- 3 Tablespoons rum
- 1 cup pumpkin puree
- 2 eggs
- ½ cup applesauce
- ⅓ cup buttermilk
- 2 Tablespoons oil
- 2 teaspoons vanilla
- Topping: hazelnuts or pecans and sugar

1. Preheat oven to 350 degrees F.
2. Pour the rum over the dates as you mix the dry ingredients.
3. Add wet ingredients, including the date-mixture, stirring just to combine (avoid overmixing).
4. Spoon batter into muffin cups, and sprinkle with nuts and sugar.
5. Bake 15-18 minutes. (Important not to overbake these). Makes 12 muffins.

Per Muffin

Calories: 223
Fat: 5g
Cholesterol: 31mg
Sodium: 163mg

Potassium: 135mg
Carbs: 40g
Fiber: 3g
Sugars: 23g
Protein: 5g

Vitamin A: 43%
Vitamin C: 9%
Calcium: 49%
Iron: 6%

Pumpkin Streusel Muffins

½ cup white whole wheat flour
½ whole wheat flour
¾ cup white flour
½ cup honey
1 Tablespoon baking powder
⅛ teaspoon salt
1 teaspoon cinnamon
½ teaspoon ginger
¼ teaspoon allspice
½ teaspoon cardamom
2 Tablespoons oil
1 cup canned pumpkin
½ cup milk
1 egg

This moist, spicy muffin is my son's favorite, and one of the few ways I got him to eat a vegetable as a boy.

1. Preheat the oven to 350 degrees F.
2. In a small bowl, prepare the streusel topping, below. Set aside.
3. In a medium bowl, mix together the dry ingredients.
4. Make a well in the middle and add the wet ingredients.
5. Stir just to combine (avoid overmixing). Spoon batter into muffin cups.
6. With your fingers, crumble the streusel topping onto each muffin. Bake 16-20 minutes. (Best if a bit underbaked.) Makes 12 muffins.
7. Variation: They're also good without the streusel topping, sprinkled with pecans and sugar, but with streusel it's a whole different experience.

Streusel Topping:
3 Tablespoons white flour
⅓ cup brown sugar
½ teaspoon cinnamon
4 teaspoons softened butter

1. Mix dry ingredients.
2. Rub in the butter until the mixture clumps together.
3. This is a basic streusel recipe that you can use with many of the muffins in this book.

Per Serving (Streusel)

Calories: 36
Fat: 1g
Cholesterol: 3mg
Sodium: 2mg
Potassium: 2mg
Carbs: 6g
Fiber: 0g
Sugars: 6g
Protein: 0g
Vitamin A: 1%
Vitamin C: 0%
Calcium: 1%
Iron: 1%

Per Muffin

Calories: 143
Fat: 3g
Cholesterol: 16mg
Sodium: 154mg
Potassium: 30mg
Carbs: 27g
Fiber: 2g
Sugars: 13g
Protein: 4g
Vitamin A: 51%
Vitamin C: 1%
Calcium: 12%
Iron: 5%

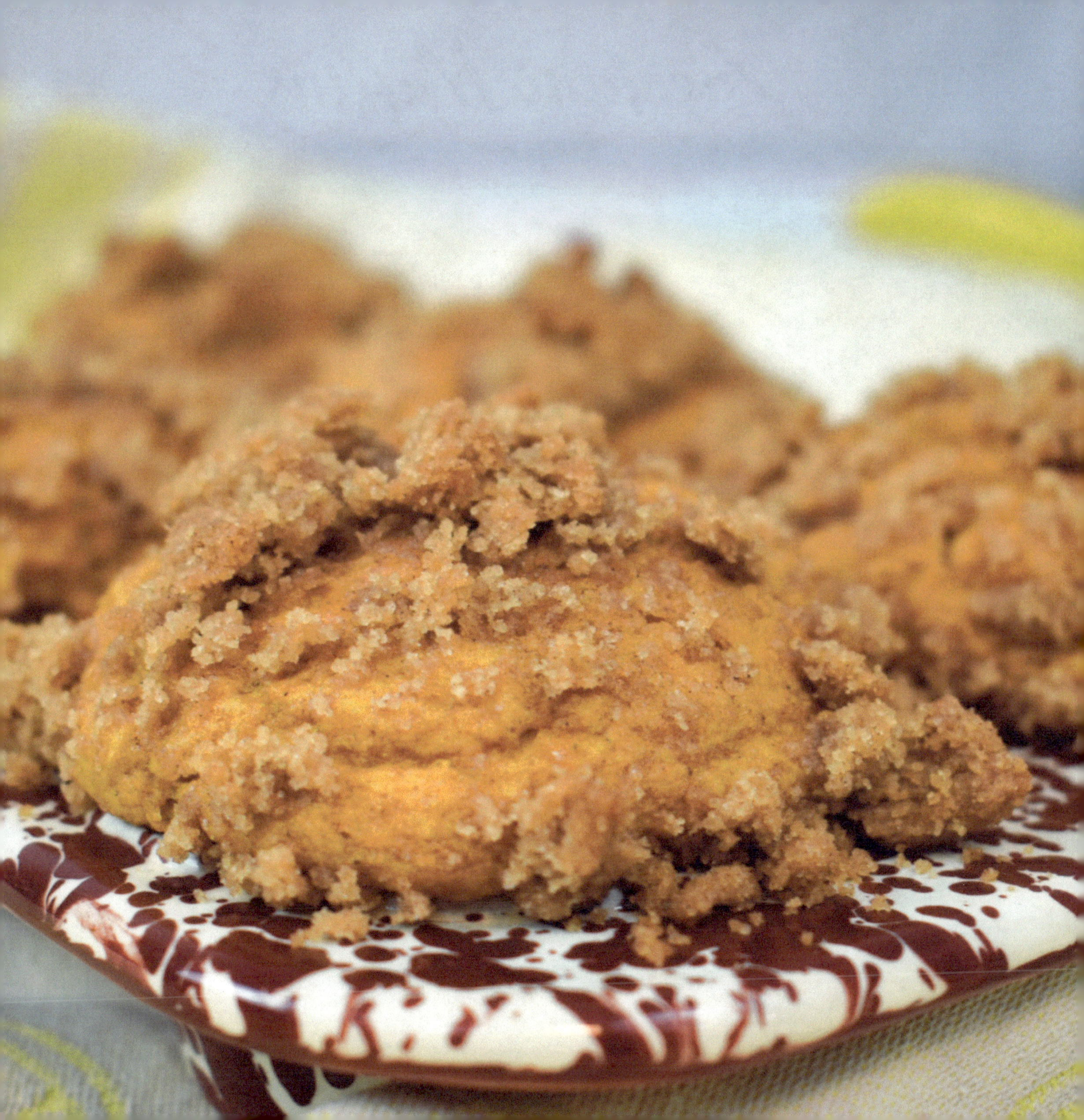

Zucchini Muffins

1 cup whole wheat flour
½ cup white flour
½ cup white whole wheat flour
2 Tablespoons brown sugar
1 Tablespoon baking powder
⅛ teaspoon salt
1 teaspoon cinnamon
⅛ teaspoon nutmeg
⅛ teaspoon cloves
⅛ teaspoon ginger
¼ cup oil
½ cup honey
2 eggs
1 teaspoon vanilla
¼ cup applesauce
1 ½ cups shredded zucchini
Topping: chopped pecans or walnuts and cinnamon sugar for sprinkling.

Even people who avoid zucchini will love these muffins, which are loaded with squash.

1. Preheat oven to 350 degrees F.
2. Combine the dry ingredients.
3. Add wet ingredients and shredded zucchini, stirring just to combine.
4. Spoon batter into muffin cups.
5. Sprinkle with nuts and cinnamon sugar.
6. Bake 15-18 minutes. (Best if a bit underbaked.)
   Makes 12 muffins.

Per Muffin

Calories: 161
Fat: 6g
Cholesterol: 26mg
Sodium: 136mg
Potassium: 21mg
Carbs: 25g
Fiber: 2g
Sugars: 12g
Protein: 3g
Vitamin A: 1%
Vitamin C: 4%
Calcium: 62%
Iron: 2%

Pumpkin Pie Muffins

You'll be tempted to top these with whipped cream when you try them.

½ cup whole wheat flour
½ cup white whole wheat flour
1 cup white flour
1 ½ teaspoons baking powder
¼ teaspoons baking soda
⅛ teaspoon salt
1 teaspoon cinnamon
½ teaspoon ginger
¼ teaspoon cloves
⅛ teaspoon nutmeg
1 cup canned pumpkin
3 Tablespoons oil
½ cup honey
¼ cup buttermilk
2 eggs
3 Tablespoons molasses
1 teaspoon vanilla
½ cup chopped dates
Topping: Walnuts and cinnamon sugar for sprinkling

1. Preheat oven to 350 degrees F.
2. Mix together dry ingredients. Rub the chopped dates into the dry ingredients to prevent clumping.
3. Add wet ingredients, stirring just to combine (best not to overmix).
4. Spoon batter into muffin cups, and sprinkle with walnuts and cinnamon sugar.
5. Bake 15-18 minutes. (Best if slightly underbaked.) Makes 12 muffins

Per Muffin

Calories: 224
Fat: 5g
Cholesterol: 31mg
Sodium: 62mg

Potassium: 153mg
Carbs: 41g
Fiber: 3g
Sugars: 24g
Protein: 4g

Vitamin A: 43%
Vitamin C: 1%
Calcium: 7%
Iron: 6%

Carrot Cake Muffins

1 cup white whole wheat flour
1 cup white flour
2 Tablespoons brown sugar
1 teaspoon baking powder
½ teaspoon baking soda
⅛ teaspoon salt
1 teaspoon cinnamon
Dash ground mace
⅓ cup applesauce
3 Tablespoons oil
½ cup honey
1 egg
1 ½ teaspoons vanilla
2 cups grated carrots
½ cup raisins
¼ cup apple juice
Topping: Cinnamon sugar and pecans for sprinkling

These muffins are seriously carroty, and the raisins, applesauce, and apple juice make them plenty sweet.

1. Preheat oven to 350 degrees F.
2. In a small bowl, soak the raisins in boiling water.
3. Meanwhile, mix together the dry ingredients.
4. Drain the raisins thoroughly.
5. Add wet ingredients, along with the raisins, stirring just to combine (careful not to overmix).
6. Spoon batter into muffin cups, and sprinkle with pecans and sugar.
7. Bake 15-18 minutes. (Always best not to overbake these). Makes 12 muffins.

Per Muffin

Calories: 200
Fat: 5g
Cholesterol: 15mg
Sodium: 126mg

Potassium: 143mg
Carbs: 36g
Fiber: 2g
Sugars: 23g
Protein: 4g

Vitamin A: 179%
Vitamin C: 10%
Calcium: 34%
Iron: 4%

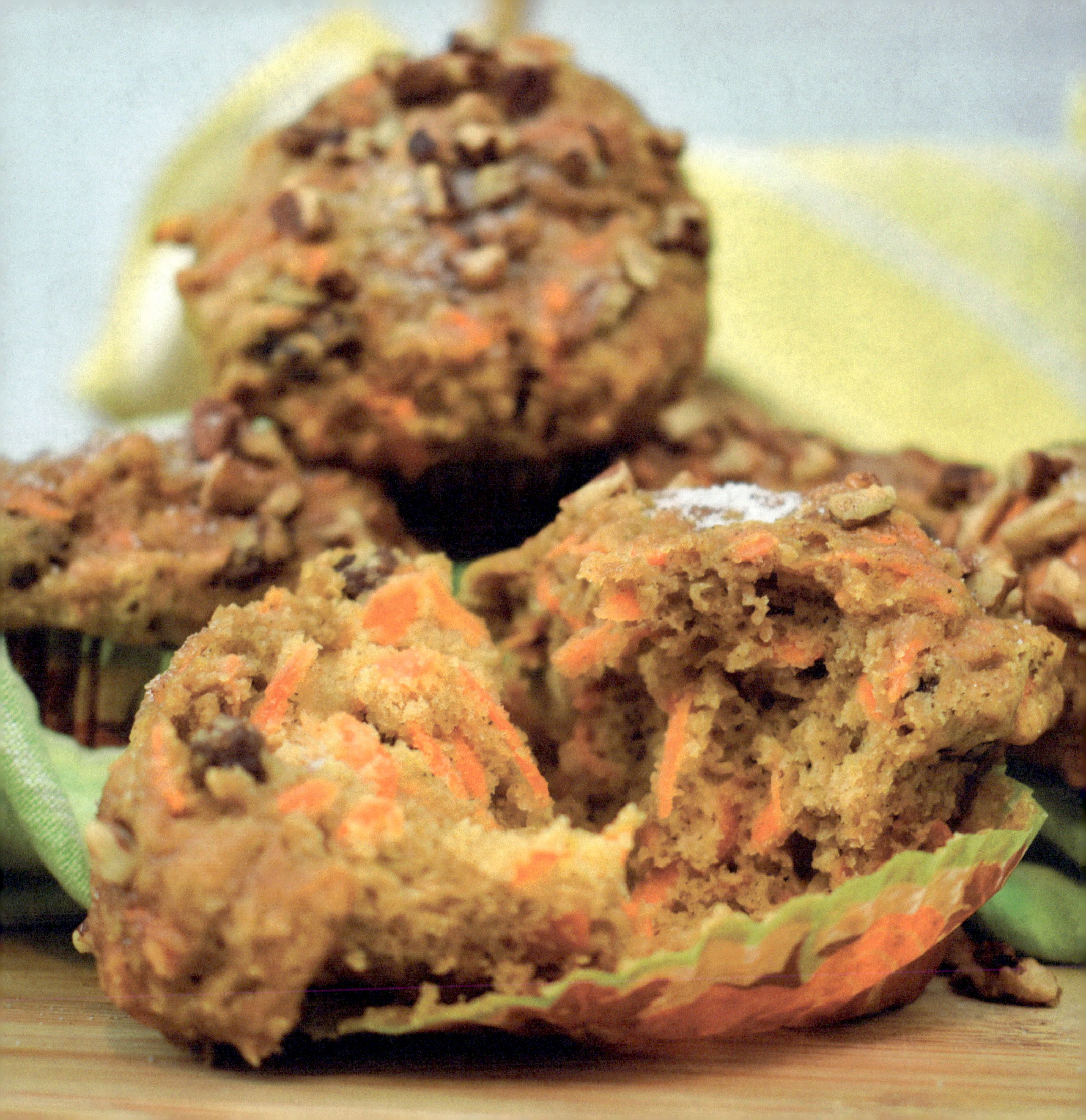

Sweet Potato Prune Muffins

½ cup white whole wheat flour
½ cup whole wheat flour
¾ cup white flour
1 Tablespoon baking powder
⅛ teaspoon salt
1 teaspoon cinnamon
½ teaspoon ginger
pinch cloves
2 Tablespoons wheat germ
1 egg
½ cup honey
1 cup mashed, cooked sweet potato
½ cup milk
2 Tablespoons oil
⅓ cup chopped prunes
Topping: Cinnamon sugar for sprinking.

A great way to use leftover baked sweet potatoes.

1. Preheat oven to 350 degrees F.
2. In a medium bowl, mix together the dry ingredients.
3. Add chopped prunes into dry ingredients and rub into the flour mixture (this will prevent clumping).
4. Make a well in the center and add wet ingredients, including the sweet potato.
5. Stir just to combine (avoid overmixing).
6. Spoon batter into muffin cups and sprinkle with cinnamon sugar.
7. Bake for 15-18 minutes. (Always best when not overbaked.) Makes 12 muffins.

Per Muffin

Calories: 162
Fat: 3g
Cholesterol: 16mg
Sodium: 164mg
Potassium: 109mg
Carbs: 30g
Fiber: 2g
Sugars: 14g
Protein: 4g
Vitamin A: 85%
Vitamin C: 0%
Calcium: 87%
Iron: 4%

Chapter 2

Seeds and Nuts for Strength

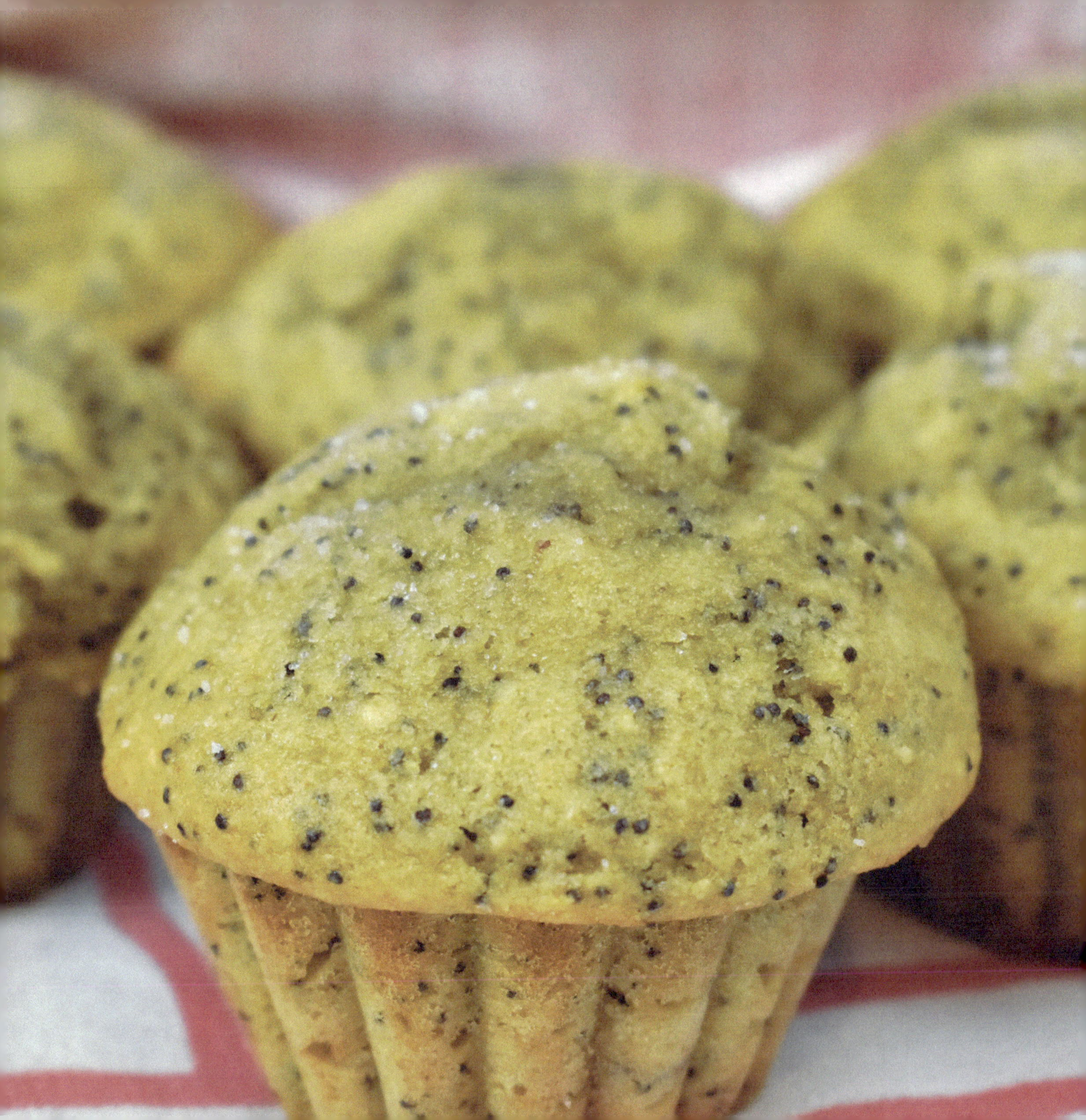

Whole Grain Sunflower Muffins

½ cup whole wheat flour
½ cup white whole wheat flour
1 cup white flour
¼ cup brown sugar
½ cup sunflower seeds
⅓ cup wheat germ
1 teaspoon baking powder
½ teaspoon baking soda
½ teaspoon salt
½ cup honey
1 cup applesauce
1 ¼ cup buttermilk
3 Tablespoons oil
1 egg
Topping: more sunflower seeds and sugar for sprinkling.

A modest yet surprisingly restorative muffin, I got the inspiration for these muffins on a visit to an elegant, old spa.

1. Preheat oven to 350 degrees F.
2. Mix together the dry ingredients.
3. Add the wet ingredients, along with the sunflower seeds, stirring just to combine (avoid overmixing).
4. Spoon batter into muffin cups, and sprinkle with sunflower seeds.
5. Bake 15-18 minutes. (Best when a bit underbaked.) Makes 12-14 muffins.
6. (If you only have a 12 cup-capacity muffin pan, bake extra batter into a mini bundt pan, or mini pie pan.)

Per Muffin

Calories: 201
Fat: 7g
Cholesterol: 17mg
Sodium: 118mg
Potassium: 86mg
Carbs: 31g
Fiber: 3g
Sugars: 16g
Protein: 5g
Vitamin A: 3%
Vitamin C: 15%
Calcium: 27%
Iron: 3%

Prune Almond Muffins

Each time I make these muffins, I wonder why I don't make them more often. Prunes and almonds make perfect companions.

- 1 cup white whole wheat flour
- 1 cup white flour
- 1 ½ teaspoons baking powder
- ½ teaspoon baking soda
- ⅛ teaspoon salt
- ½ cup honey with a bit of molasses
- 1 teaspoon vanilla
- ¼ teaspoon almond extract
- ½ cup sour cream
- ¼ cup butter, melted and cooled
- ¼ cup applesauce
- 1 cup chopped, stewed prunes
- ¼ cup buttermilk
- 2 eggs
- Topping: chopped almonds and sugar

1. Preheat oven to 350 degrees F.
2. With a fork, pick out the prunes and chop them coarsely.
3. Mix together the dry ingredients.
4. As you measure the honey, just before you reach the top of the measure, top it off with molasses (2-3 tablespoons worth).
5. Add wet ingredients, along with the prunes, stirring just to combine.
6. Spoon batter into muffin cups, and sprinkle with almonds and sugar.
7. Bake 15-18 minutes. (Always best slightly underbaked.) Makes 12 muffins.
8. Note: I stew the prunes the night before so they get nice and plump.

Per Muffin

Calories: 179
Fat: 7g
Cholesterol: 45mg
Sodium: 89mg

Potassium: 148mg
Carbs: 26g
Fiber: 2g
Sugars: 16g
Protein: 4g

Vitamin A: 36%
Vitamin C: 4%
Calcium: 11%
Iron: 2%

Silk Road Muffins

½ cup whole wheat flour
½ cup white whole wheat flour
¾ cup white flour
⅛ teaspoon salt
1 Tablespoon baking powder
¾ teaspoon cardamom
½ cup honey
¼ cup brown sugar
½ cup milk
¼ cup tahini (ground sesame)
½ teaspoon Asian sesame oil
½ teaspoon salt
2 Tablespoons oil
⅓ cup applesauce
1 egg
½ cup chopped dates
Topping: Sesame seeds and sugar for sprinkling.

An evocative muffin with the flavors of the Near East. My personal favorite.

1. Preheat oven to 350 degrees F.
2. Mix the dry ingredients together.
3. Add the chopped dates into the dry ingredients and rub them into the flour with your fingers (this will prevent clumping).
4. In a separate bowl, mix honey and tahini until it forms a paste.
5. Add other wet ingredients into the tahini mixture, then stir this into the dry mixture until just blended (avoid overmixing).
6. Spoon batter into muffin cups and sprinkle each with sesame seeds, followed by sugar.
7. Bake for 16-20 minutes (with these, it's important not to over-bake). Makes 12 muffins.

Per Muffin

Calories: 232
Fat: 7g
Cholesterol: 16mg
Sodium: 257mg

Potassium: 123mg
Carbs: 40g
Fiber: 2g
Sugars: 26g
Protein: 5g

Vitamin A: 4%
Vitamin C: 86%
Calcium: 11%
Iron: 3%

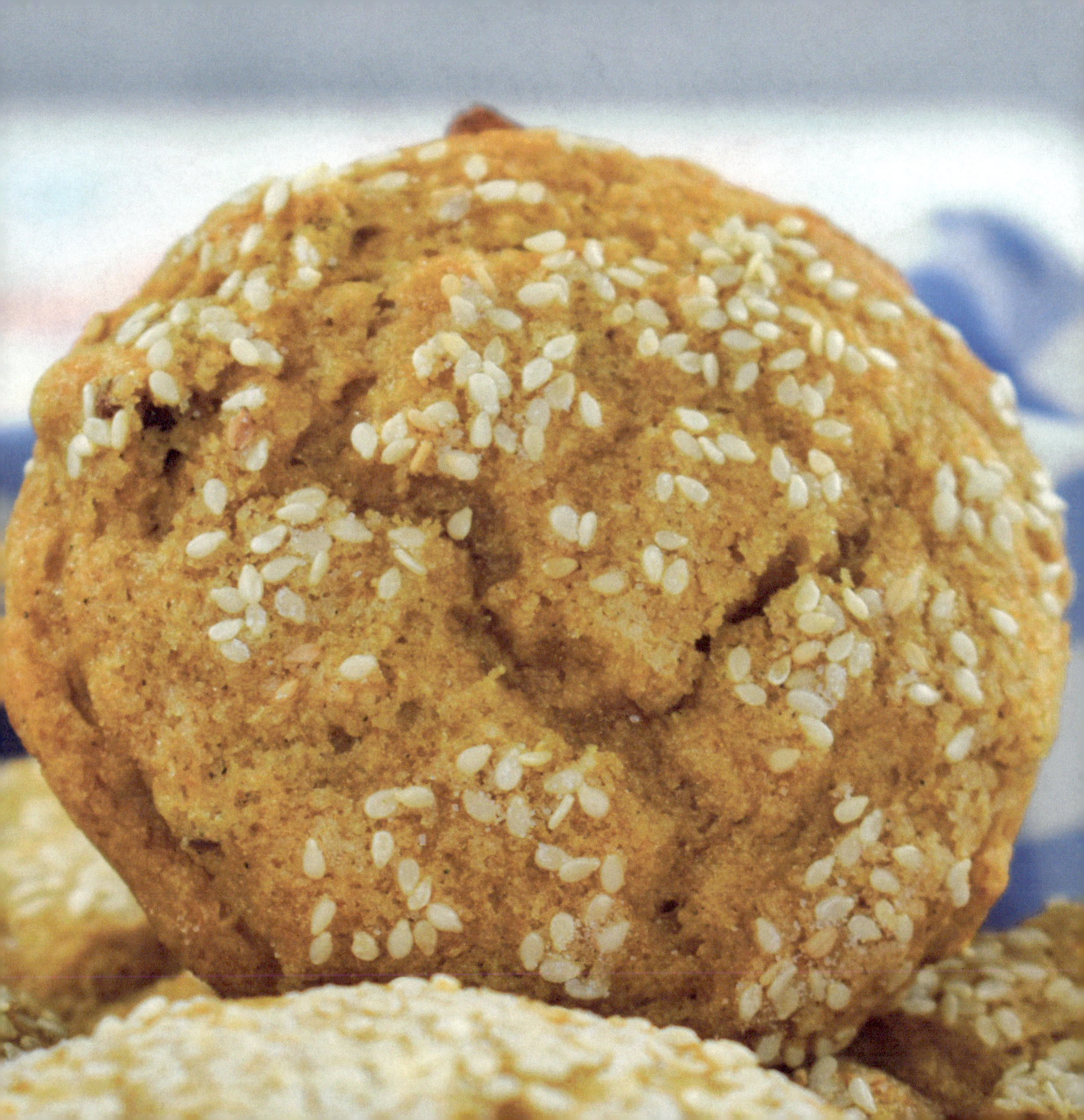

Carrot Tahini Muffins

2 Tablespoons oil
¼ cup tahini
½ cup honey
2 Tablespoons brown sugar
2 eggs
¾ cup buttermilk
1 teaspoon vanilla-orange extract blend
½ teaspoon baking soda
⅛ teaspoon salt
1 cup white whole wheat flour
1 cup white flour
2 teaspoons baking powder
2 cups grated carrots

Glaze:
¼ cup powdered sugar
3 Tablespoons tahini
2 Tablespoons water

With or without the glaze, these carroty muffins are so satisfying.

1. Preheat oven to 350 degrees F.
2. Mix together oil, tahini, eggs, honey, brown sugar, and extract.
3. Combine the dry ingredients and add to the wet ingredients alternately with buttermilk, then shredded carrots, stirring just to combine.
4. Spoon batter into muffin cups.
5. Bake 15-18 minutes. (Best if not overbaked.)
6. While muffins bake, make the glaze topping, stirring until smooth.
7. Cool muffins slightly and spread glaze on muffins. Makes 12-14 muffins.
8. (If you only have a 12 cup-capacity muffin pan, bake extra batter into a mini bundt pan, or mini pie pan.)

Per Muffin

Calories: 200
Fat: 6g
Cholesterol: 31mg
Sodium: 185mg
Potassium: 111mg
Carbs: 32g
Fiber: 2g
Sugars: 15g
Protein: 5g
Vitamin A: 179%
Vitamin C: 2%
Calcium: %
Iron: 4%

Per Glaze Serving

Calories: 34
Fat: 2g
Cholesterol: 0mg
Sodium: 0mg
Potassium: 0mg
Carbs: 4g
Fiber: 1g
Sugars: 3g
Protein: 1g
Vitamin A: 0%
Vitamin C: 0%
Calcium: 0%
Iron: 0%

Peanut Butter Muffins

A wonderfully substantial muffin with a note of ginger.

- ½ cup whole wheat flour
- ½ cup white whole wheat flour
- ⅔ cup white flour
- ⅛ teaspoon salt
- 1 Tablespoon baking powder
- ½ teaspoon ginger
- ½ cup honey
- ½ cup milk
- ½ cup peanut butter
- ⅓ cup applesauce
- 2 Tablespoons oil
- 1 egg
- 1 ½ teaspoons vanilla

1. Preheat oven to 350 degrees F.
2. In a medium bowl, blend peanut butter and honey until smooth.
3. Add eggs, oil, milk, vanilla and applesauce.
4. In a separate bowl, sift together the dry ingredients, and combine with the wet ingredients.
5. Spoon batter into muffin cups.
6. Bake for 15-18 minutes. Makes 12 muffins.
7. Variation: Why not add 1/2 cup of semi-sweet chocolate chips?

Per Muffin

Calories: 195
Fat: 8g
Cholesterol: 16mg
Sodium: 192mg

Potassium: 33mg
Carbs: 27g
Fiber: 2g
Sugars: 14g
Protein: 5g

Vitamin A: 3%
Vitamin C: 6%
Calcium: 82%
Iron: 4%

Lemon Poppy Seed Muffins

1 ½ cups white whole wheat flour
½ cup white flour
⅛ teaspoon salt
½ cup honey
½ teaspoon baking soda
3 Tablespoons poppy seeds
½ cup low-fat sour cream
2 eggs
½ teaspoon vanilla
Grated rind of one organic lemon
½ cup applesauce
2 Tablespoons oil
2 Tablespoons milk
Topping: white sugar for sprinkling

I know without even asking what kind of muffin my husband would like in the morning. These!

1. Preheat oven to 350 degrees F.
2. In a medium bowl, mix together the dry ingredients.
3. Grate the lemon rind directly over the bowl so as not to lose the oils.
4. Make a well in the center and add the wet ingredients.
5. Stir just to combine (avoid overmixing).
6. Spoon batter into muffin cups. Sprinkle white sugar over muffins.
7. Bake for 16-20 minutes. (Best if a bit underbaked.) Makes 12 muffins.

Per Muffin

Calories: 173
Fat: 5g
Cholesterol: 34mg
Sodium: 87mg
Potassium: 63mg
Carbs: 27g
Fiber: 2g
Sugars: 14g
Protein: 5g
Vitamin A: 16%
Vitamin C: 8%
Calcium: 9%
Iron: 4%

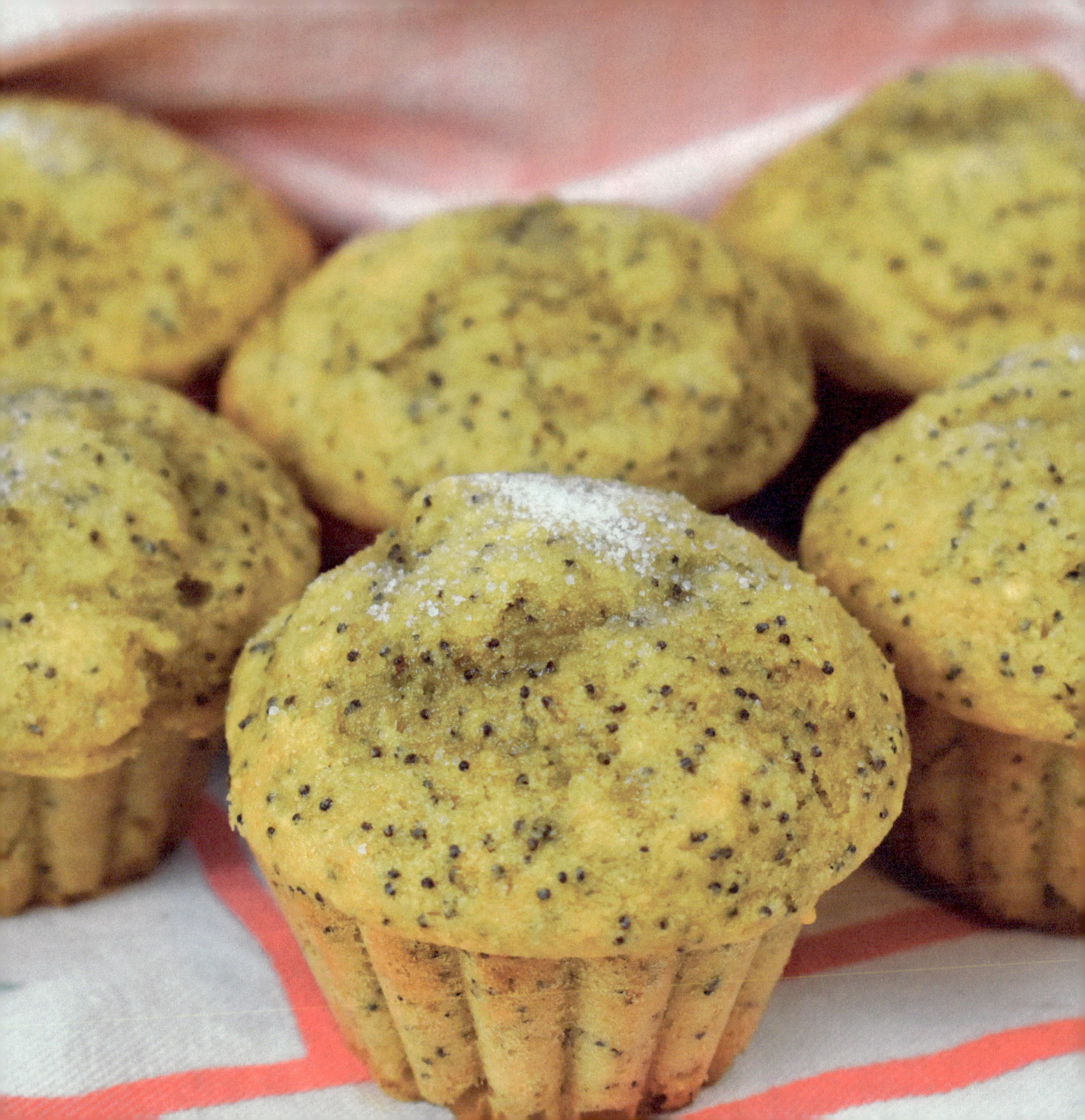

Chapter 3
Chocolate for Good Cheer

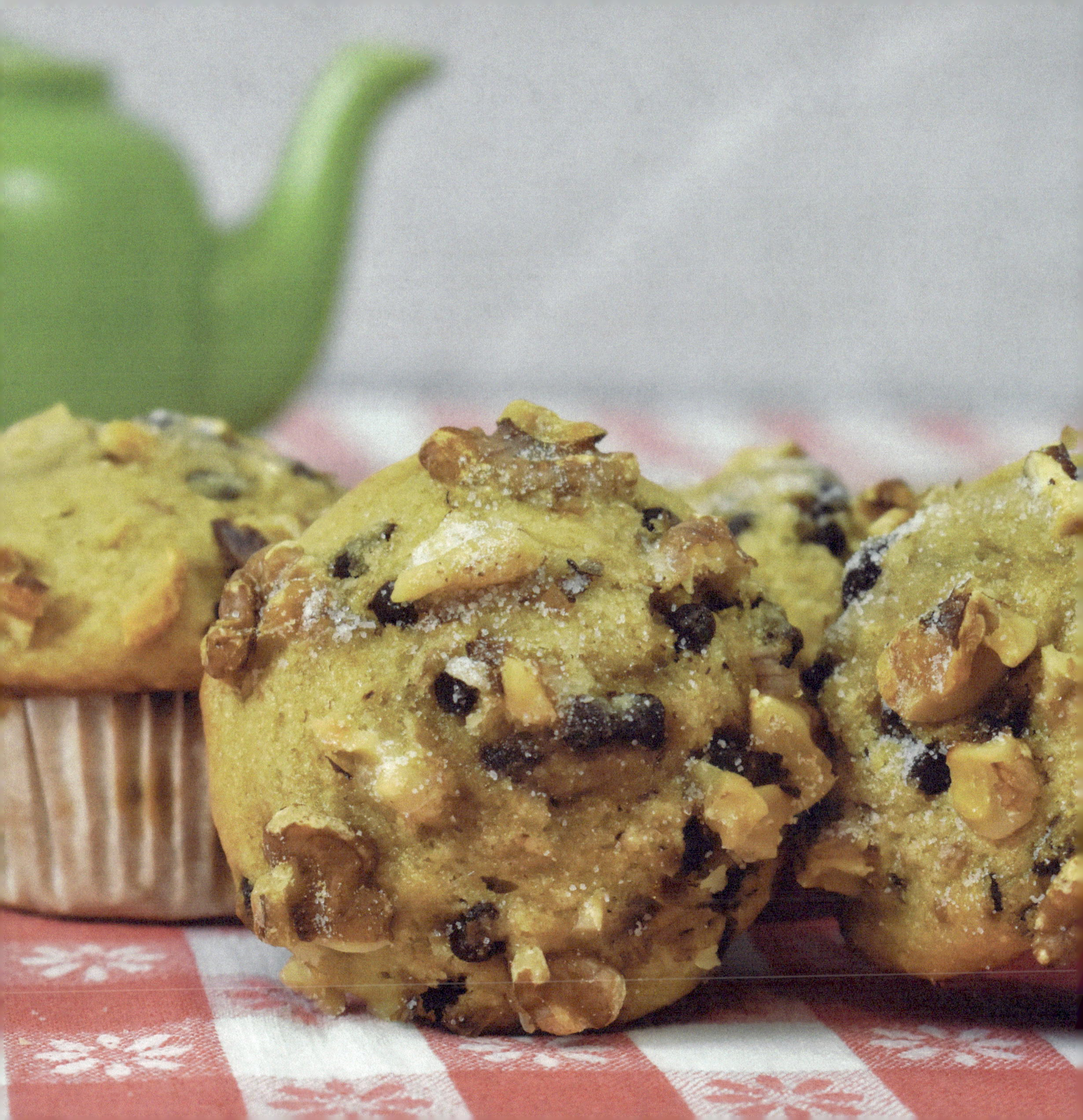

Black Forest Muffins

½ cup whole wheat flour
½ cup white whole wheat flour
1 cup white flour
1 Tablespoon baking powder
3 Tablespoons cocoa powder
⅛ teaspoon salt
½ cup applesauce
1 teaspoon vanilla
2 Tablespoons oil
⅔ cup milk
½ cup honey
1 egg
½ cup mini semi-sweet chocolate chips
½ cup dried cherries, chopped
Topping: Sugar for sprinkling.

I make these when we have something to celebrate, or simply feel like indulging.

1. Preheat oven to 350 degrees F.
2. Mix together the dry ingredients.
3. Stir the dried cherries into the dry ingredients (to prevent clumping later).
4. Make a well in the center and add the wet ingredients along with chocolate chips, stirring just to combine (avoid overmixing).
5. Spoon batter into muffin cups and sprinkle with sugar.
6. Bake for 15-20 minutes. (Important not to overbake these.) Makes 12 muffins.
7. Variation: Top with your favorite nuts.

Per Muffin

Calories: 224
Fat: 6g
Cholesterol: 17mg
Sodium: 161mg
Potassium: 59mg
Carbs: 40g
Fiber: 3g
Sugars: 23g
Protein: 6g
Vitamin A: 4%
Vitamin C: 0%
Calcium: 87%
Iron: 3%

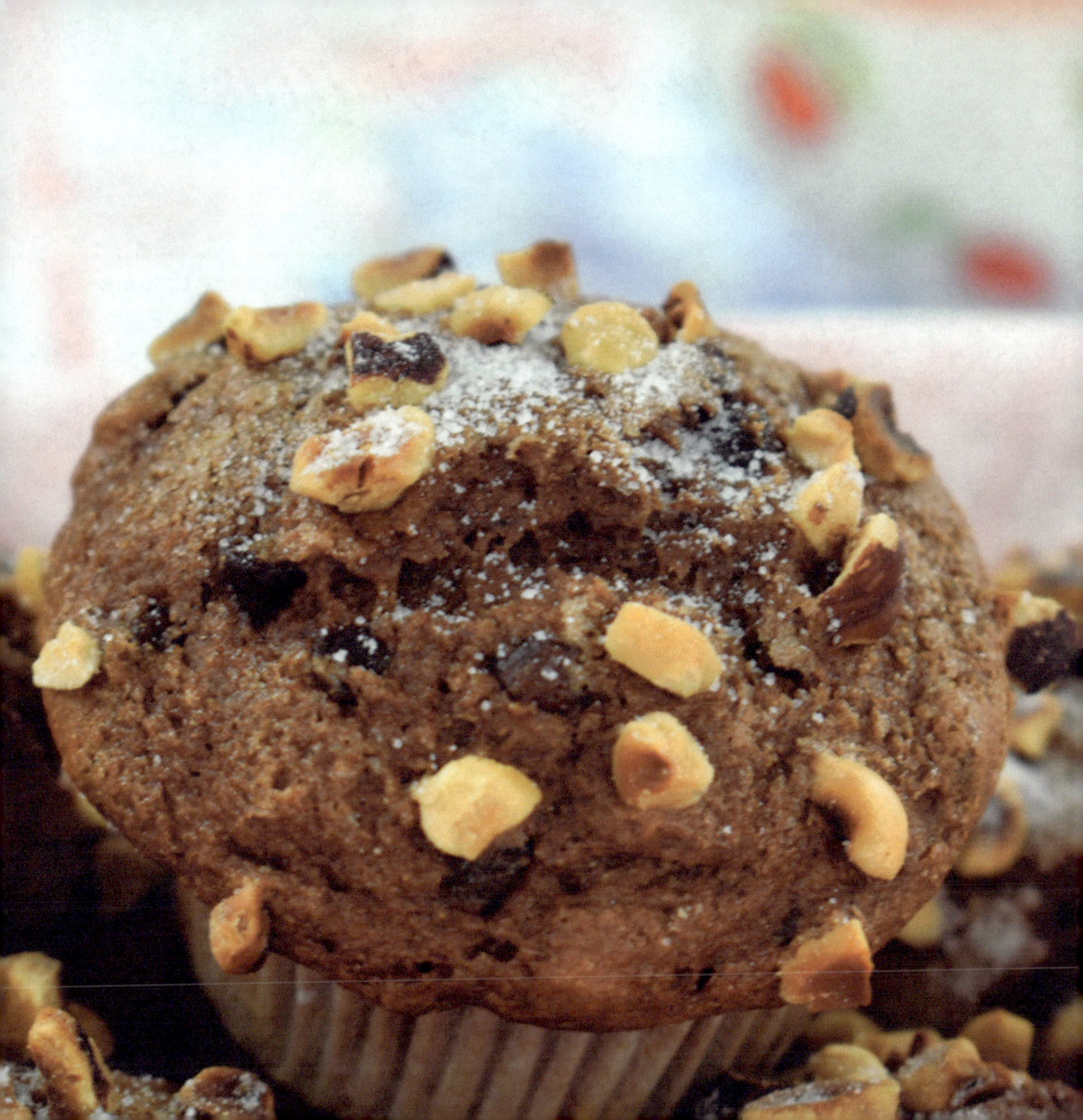

Mocha Chip Muffins

½ cup white whole wheat flour
½ cup whole wheat flour
1 cup white flour
½ teaspoon baking soda
⅛ teaspoon salt
½ cup honey
¼ cup brown sugar
¼ cup powdered coffee dissolved in 2 Tablespoons of water
⅔ cup applesauce
1 egg
½ cup buttermilk
1 teaspoon vanilla
2 Tablespoons oil
½ cup mini semi-sweet chocolate chips
Topping: sugar for sprinkling.

After these muffins, you can face any day.

1. Preheat oven to 350 degrees F.
2. In a medium bowl, mix together the dry ingredients.
3. Make a well in the center and add the wet ingredients along with chocolate chips.
4. Stir just to combine (avoid overmixing).
5. Spoon batter into muffin cups. Sprinkle with sugar.
6. Bake for 15-18 minutes. (Best if a bit underbaked.) Makes 12 muffins.

Per Muffin

Calories: 219
Fat: 6g
Cholesterol: 16mg
Sodium: 86mg

Potassium: 29mg
Carbs: 39g
Fiber: 2g
Sugars: 24g
Protein: 4g

Vitamin A: 1%
Vitamin C: 11%
Calcium: 7%
Iron: 2%

Malted Milk Muffins

The malt powder in these makes them mysteriously good.

1 cup white whole wheat flour
¾ cup white flour
1 Tablespoon baking powder
½ cup malted milk powder
⅛ teaspoon salt
½ cup honey
⅓ cup applesauce
2 Tablespoons oil
¾ cup buttermilk
1 egg
½ teaspoon vanilla
⅓ cup mini semi-sweet chocolate chips
Topping: slivered almonds and sugar

1. Preheat oven to 350 degrees F.
2. Mix together the dry ingredients.
3. Add the wet ingredients, stirring just to combine (avoid overmixing).
4. Spoon batter into muffin cups, and sprinkle with almonds and sugar.
5. Bake 15-18 minutes. (Always best not to overbake). Makes 12 muffins.
6. Variation: For chocolate malt muffins, add 2 Tablespoons cocoa powder into the dry ingredients, or subsitute chocolate malt powder for plain malt powder.

Per Muffin

Calories: 203
Fat: 6g
Cholesterol: 17mg
Sodium: 209mg
Potassium: 41mg
Carbs: 33g
Fiber: 2g
Sugars: 18g
Protein: 4g
Vitamin A: 1%
Vitamin C: 6%
Calcium: 72%
Iron: 3%

Chocolate Chip Muffins

½ cup whole wheat flour
½ cup white whole wheat flour
1 cup white flour
⅛ teaspoon salt
½ cup honey
2 teaspoons baking powder
½ cup milk
½ cup applesauce
2 Tablespoons oil
2 eggs
1 teaspoon vanilla
¾ cup mini semi-sweet chocolate chips
Topping: ½ cup walnuts (optional), and white sugar for sprinkling.

Healthy and decadent all in one.

1. Preheat oven to 350 degrees F.
2. In a medium bowl, mix together the dry ingredients.
3. Make a well in the center and add wet ingredients and the chocolate chips.
4. Stir just to combine (avoid overmixing).
5. Spoon batter into muffin cups.
6. Sprinkle with walnuts, if desired, followed by sugar.
7. Bake for 18-20 minutes. (Like the cookie version, best if a bit underbaked. Makes 12 muffins.

Per Muffin

Calories: 260
Fat: 6g
Cholesterol: 32mg
Sodium: 125mg

Potassium: 62mg
Carbs: 38g
Fiber: 3g
Sugars: 22g
Protein: 5g

Vitamin A: 16%
Vitamin C: 8%
Calcium: 68%
Iron: 2%

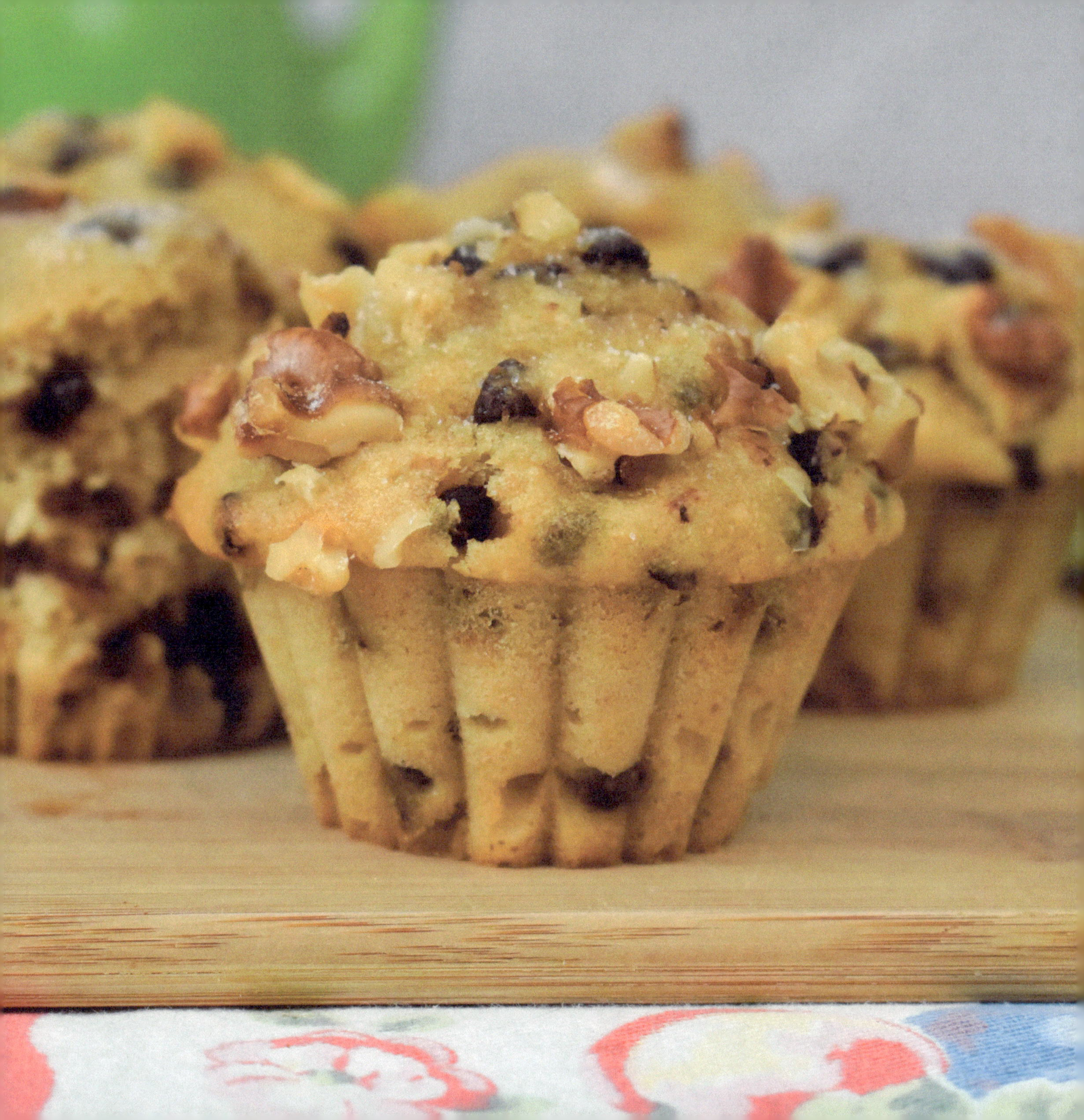

Chapter 4
Berries for Beauty

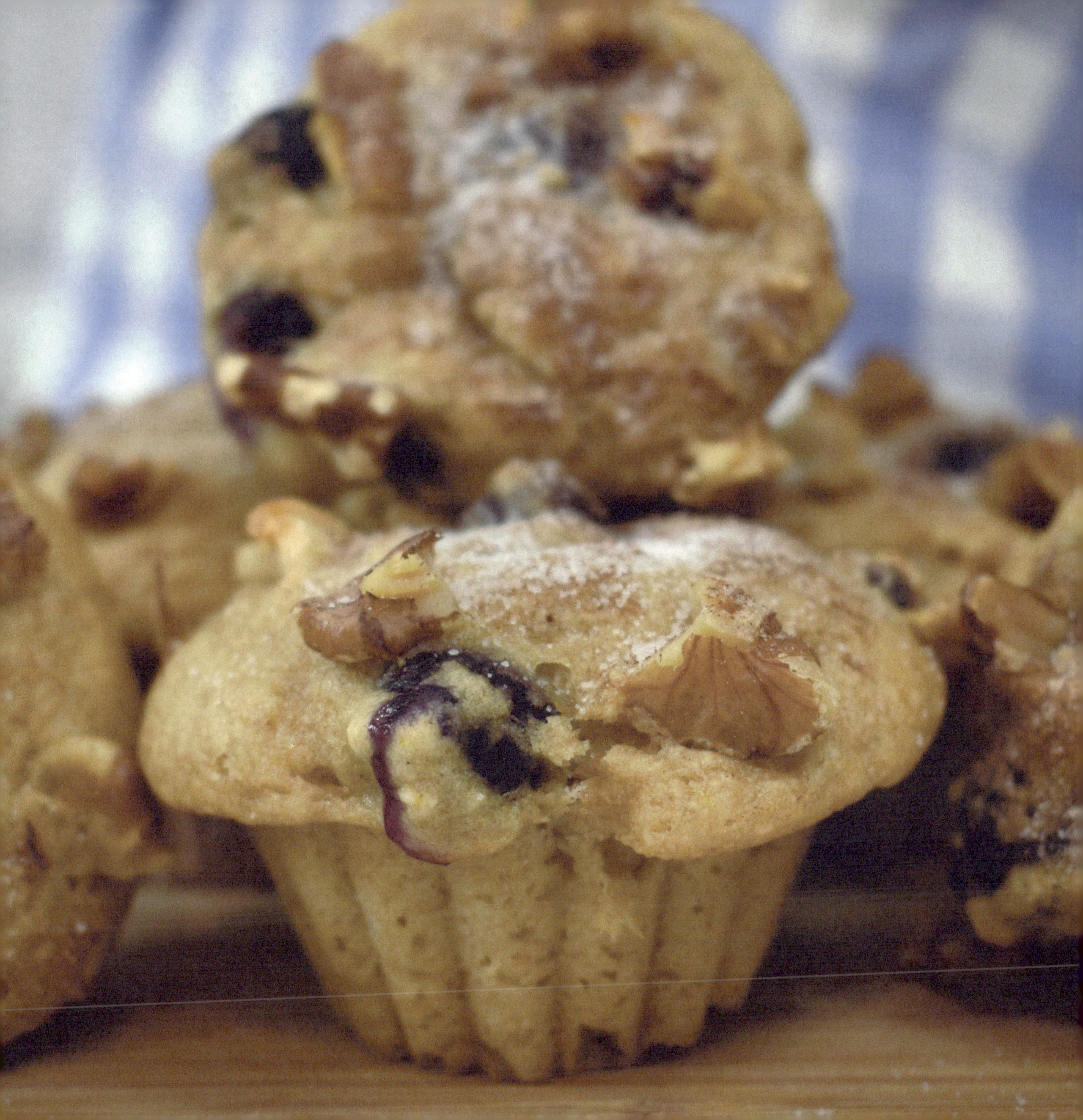

Strawberry Lemon Muffins

1 cup white whole wheat flour
¾ cup white flour
⅛ teaspoon salt
1 teaspoon baking soda
½ cup honey
⅓ cup applesauce
Zest from one lemon
2 teaspoons fresh lemon juice
2 eggs
3 Tablespoons oil
½ teaspoon vanilla
2 cups fresh strawberries, finely chopped

Crumb Topping:
⅓ cup brown sugar
3 Tablespoons flour
4 teaspoons butter

I started making these during strawberry season, and now they're specially requested

1. Preheat oven to 350 degrees F.
2. In a small bowl, combine the crumb topping mixture, so it's ready to go when the batter is ready.
3. Mix together the dry ingredients.
4. Add the wet ingredients, along with the chopped strawberries, stirring just to combine. (The batter will seem thick, but the berries create their own moisture.)
5. Spoon batter into muffin cups. Sprinkle with crumb topping.
6. Bake for 15-18 minutes. (Always best not to overbake.) Makes 12 muffins.

Per Muffin

Calories: 158
Fat: 5g
Cholesterol: 31mg
Sodium: 111mg
Potassium: 67mg
Carbs: 26g
Fiber: 2g
Sugars: 13g
Protein: 4g
Vitamin A: 1%
Vitamin C: 24%
Calcium: 6%
Iron: 3%

Per Crumb Topping

Calories: 36
Fat: 1g
Cholesterol: 3mg
Sodium: 2mg
Potassium: 9mg
Carbs: 6g
Fiber: 0g
Sugars: 6g
Protein: 0g
Vitamin A: 10%
Vitamin C: 0%
Calcium: 6%
Iron: 0%

Lemon-Blackberry Muffins

Tangy and sweet at the same time.

½ cup whole wheat flour
½ cup white whole wheat flour
1 cup white flour
2 teaspoons baking powder
⅛ teaspoon salt
½ cup honey
⅓ cup applesauce
Grated zest of one organic lemon
1 egg
½ cup milk
½ teaspoon vanilla
2 Tablespoons oil
1 cup blackberries, chopped slightly
Topping: Sugar for sprinkling

1. Preheat oven to 350 degrees F.
2. Mix together dry ingredients.
3. Make a well in the center and add the wet ingredients, along with the berries, stirring just to combine (avoid overmixing).
4. Spoon batter into muffin cups.
5. Sprinkle with sugar.
6. Bake for 15-18 minutes. Makes 12 muffins.

Per Muffin

Calories: 145
Fat: 4g
Cholesterol: 16mg
Sodium: 117mg
Potassium: 65mg
Carbs: 24g
Fiber: 2g
Sugars: 13g
Protein: 3g
Vitamin A: 5%
Vitamin C: 8%
Calcium: 63%
Iron: 5%

Fresh Blueberry Muffins

½ cup whole wheat flour
½ cup white whole wheat flour
1 cup white flour
⅛ teaspoon salt
1 Tablespoon baking powder
½ cup honey
½ cup milk
2 Tablespoons oil
½ cup applesauce
1 egg
2 teaspoons vanilla
1 ½ cups fresh blueberries
Topping: ½ cup chopped walnuts, and cinnamon sugar for sprinkling.

I only make these with fresh blueberries, which I pick at a local farm, a treat my family looks forward to all year.

1. Preheat oven to 350 degrees F.
2. In a medium bowl, mix together the dry ingredients. (If you're making the lemon version, grate the lemon rind directly over the bowl of dry ingredients.)
3. Make a well in the center and add the wet ingredients.
4. Stir just to combine (avoid overmixing).
5. Fold in the blueberries.
6. Spoon batter into muffin cups and sprinkle with walnuts, followed by cinnamon sugar.
7. Bake for 15-18 minutes. (Best if a bit underbaked.) Makes 12 muffins.
8. Variation: For Lemon Blueberry Muffins, reduce vanilla to ½ teaspoon, and add the grated rind of one organic lemon to batter. Sprinkle with plain white sugar.

Per Muffin

Calories: 192
Fat: 6g
Cholesterol: 16mg
Sodium: 160mg

Potassium: 67mg
Carbs: 31g
Fiber: 2g
Sugars: 14g
Protein: 4g

Vitamin A: 4%
Vitamin C: 10%
Calcium: 87%
Iron: 2%

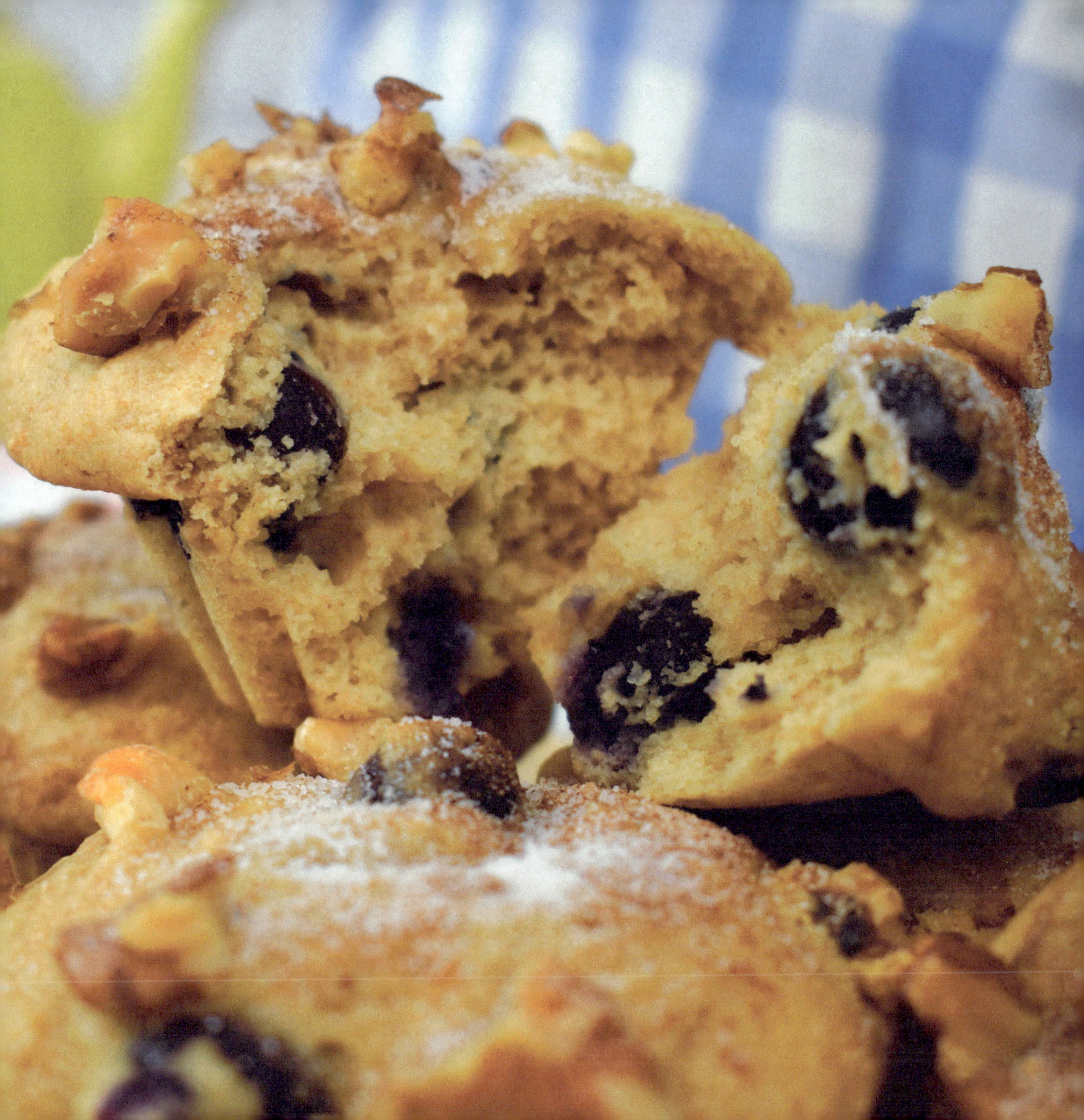

Autumn Cranberry-Nut Muffins

- 1 cup whole wheat flour
- 1 cup white flour
- ⅛ teaspoon salt
- ⅔ cup honey
- 1 ½ teaspoons baking powder
- ½ teaspoon baking soda
- 1 teaspoon cinnamon
- ¾ cup orange juice
- 2 Tablespoons oil
- 1 egg
- 1 ½ cups whole cranberries, coarsely chopped
- Topping: ½ cup chopped walnuts or pecans, cinnamon sugar

Full of cranberries and flavor!

1. Preheat oven to 350 degrees F.
2. Mix the dry ingredients together.
3. Stir in wet ingredients, followed by cranberries just until blended.
4. Spoon batter into muffin cups and sprinkle with nuts, followed by cinnamon sugar.
5. Bake for 16-18 minutes. (Best if a bit underbaked.) Makes 12 muffins.

Per Muffin

Calories: 200
Fat: 6g
Cholesterol: 16mg
Sodium: 130mg

Potassium: 80mg
Carbs: 34g
Fiber: 2g
Sugars: 18g
Protein: 4g

Vitamin A: 8%
Vitamin C: 11%
Calcium: 47%
Iron: 1%

Chapter 5
Bananas for Boldness

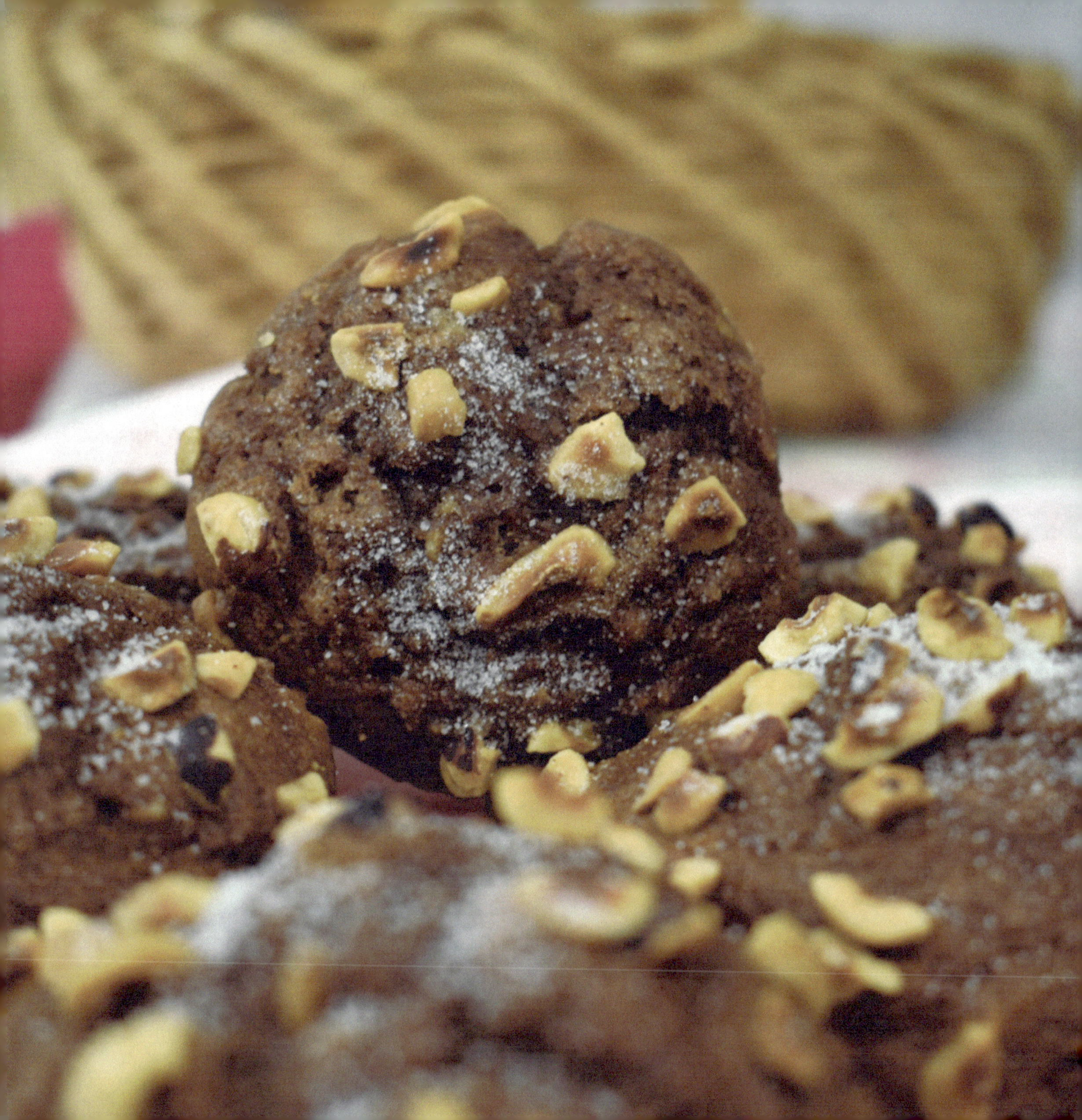

Banana Nut Muffins

- ½ cup whole wheat flour
- ¾ cup white whole wheat flour
- 1 cup white flour
- ⅛ teaspoon salt
- 1 ½ teaspoons baking powder
- 1 teaspoon baking soda
- ½ cup honey
- ½ cup milk
- 2 Tablespoons oil
- 2 teaspoons vanilla
- 2 eggs
- 3 medium ripe bananas (1 ½ cups), mashed
- Topping: sprinkle with ½ cup chopped walnuts and white sugar

Extra vanilla brightens up this classic muffin.

1. Preheat oven to 350 degrees F.
2. In a medium bowl, mix together the dry ingredients.
3. Make a well in the center and add wet ingredients.
4. Stir just to combine (avoid overmixing).
5. Spoon batter into muffin cups.
6. Sprinkle the walnuts and sugar over the tops.
7. Bake for 15-18 minutes. (Best if a bit underbaked.) Makes 12 muffins.
8. Variation: Omit walnuts and add ½ teaspoon ginger and ¼ cup chopped crystallized ginger.
9. Another Variation: Stir ½ cup mini semi-sweet chocolate chips into the batter when you add the wet ingredients

Per Muffin

Calories: 226
Fat: 7g
Cholesterol: 32mg
Sodium: 176mg

Potassium: 124mg
Carbs: 37g
Fiber: 3g
Sugars: 17g
Protein: 6g

Vitamin A: 17%
Vitamin C: 3%
Calcium: 59%
Iron: 3%

Banana Blueberry Muffins

I was skeptical of this combination until I tried it. Who knew?!

¾ cup buttermilk
½ cup honey
2 Tablespoons brown sugar
3 Tablespoons oil
1 egg
1 cup mashed bananas (about 3)
1 ¼ cups whole wheat flour
1 cup white flour
1 ½ teaspoons baking powder
¾ teaspoon cinnamon
½ teaspoon baking soda
⅛ teaspoon salt
¼ teaspoon nutmeg
1 ¼ cups fresh blueberries
Topping: Sugar for sprinkling

1. Preheat oven to 350 degrees F.
2. Mix together the dry ingredients.
3. Add wet ingredients and blueberries, gently stirring just to combine.
4. Spoon batter into muffin cups. Sprinkle with sugar.
5. Bake for 15-18 minutes. (Best when slightly underbaked.) Makes 12-14 muffins.

Per Muffin

Calories: 213
Fat: 4g
Cholesterol: 19mg
Sodium: 84mg

Potassium: 198mg
Carbs: 40g
Fiber: 3g
Sugars: 20g
Protein: 5g

Vitamin A: 2%
Vitamin C: 6%
Calcium: 6%
Iron: 2%

Cocoa-Banana Nut Muffins

½ cup whole wheat flour
½ cup white whole wheat flour
1 cup white flour
1 Tablespoon baking powder
3 Tablespoons cocoa powder
⅛ teaspoon salt
½ cup honey
2-3 ripe bananas, mashed
2 Tablespoons oil
1 teaspoon vanilla
⅔ cup milk
1 egg
Topping: Walnuts or hazelnuts, and sugar for sprinkling.

When in doubt, I make these muffins, and it's always the right choice.

1. Preheat oven to 350 degrees F.
2. Mix together the dry ingredients.
3. Make a well in the center and add the wet ingredients, stirring just to combine (avoid overmixing).
4. Spoon batter into muffin cups and sprinkle with nuts, followed by sugar.
5. Bake for 15-18 minutes. (Always best not to overbake these.) Makes 12 muffins.

Per Muffin

Calories: 183
Fat: 4g
Cholesterol: 17mg
Sodium: 159mg

Potassium: 127mg
Carbs: 33g
Fiber: 2g
Sugars: 16g
Protein: 4g

Vitamin A: 5%
Vitamin C: 4%
Calcium: 86%
Iron: 5%

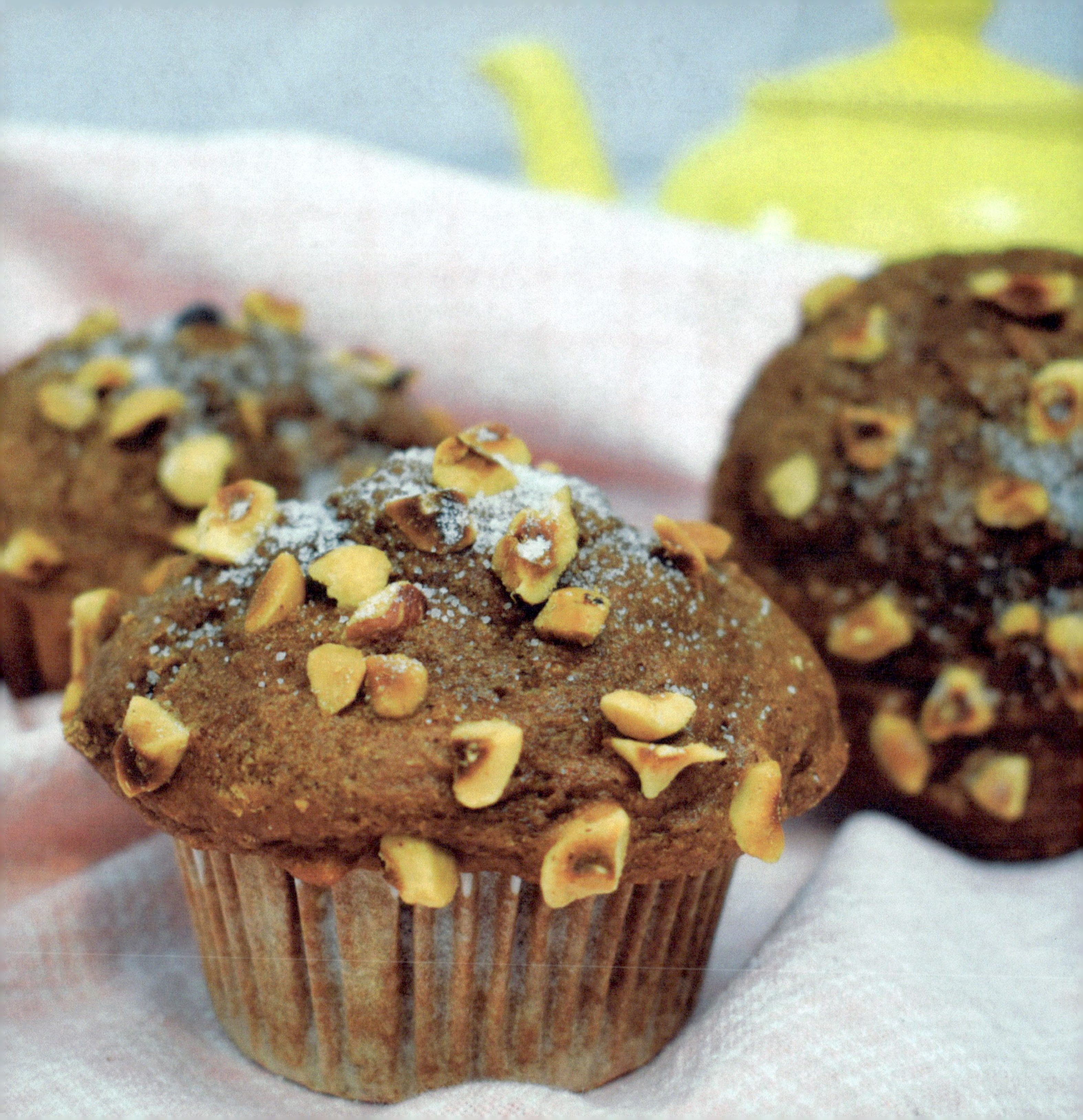

Banana Sour Cream Muffins

1 ¼ cups white whole wheat flour
1 cup white flour
2 Tablespoons brown sugar
¼ cup butter, melted
1 cup mashed bananas (about 3 bananas)
2 eggs
1 teaspoon vanilla
1 ½ teaspoons baking powder
½ teaspoons baking soda
⅛ teaspoon salt
½ cup honey
1 cup light sour cream
Topping: ½ cup walnuts or pecans and sugar for sprinkling

The sour cream in these gives them a smooth, comforting texture.

1. Preheat oven to 350 degrees F.
2. Mix together the dry ingredients.
3. Add the wet ingredients, stirring just to combine (avoid overmixing).
4. Spoon batter into muffin cups.
5. Sprinkle with sugar and nuts.
6. Bake 15-18 minutes. (Best if slightly underbaked.) Makes 12 muffins.

Per Muffin

Calories: 238
Fat: 7g
Cholesterol: 48mg
Sodium: 54mg

Potassium: 181mg
Carbs: 38g
Fiber: 2g
Sugars: 19g
Protein: 6g

Vitamin A: 36%
Vitamin C: 5%
Calcium: 7%
Iron: 5%

Peanut Butter Banana Muffins

A healthy, nutritious muffin and kid favorite.

1. Preheat oven to 350 degrees F.
2. Blend together the honey, peanut butter, and brown sugar in a small bowl.
3. Combine the dry ingredients, and add all the remaining ingredients, including the honey mixture, stirring just to combine.
4. Spoon batter into muffin cups, and sprinkle with sugar.
5. Bake 15-18 minutes. (Best when a bit underbaked.) Makes 12 muffins.

½ cup whole wheat flour
¾ cup white whole wheat flour
1 cup white flour
1 teaspoon baking powder
1 teaspoon baking soda
½ cup honey
⅓ cup creamy peanut butter
2 Tablespoons brown sugar
¼ cup applesauce
3 bananas mashed
2 Tablespoons oil
2 eggs
1 ½ teaspoons vanilla
⅓ cup sour cream
Topping: Sugar for sprinkling

Per Muffin

Calories: 246
Fat: 7g
Cholesterol: 33mg
Sodium: 156mg

Potassium: 135mg
Carbs: 39g
Fiber: 3g
Sugars: 19g
Protein: 7g

Vitamin A: 2%
Vitamin C: 9%
Calcium: 26%
Iron: 4%

Chapter 6

Apples and Apricots for Agility

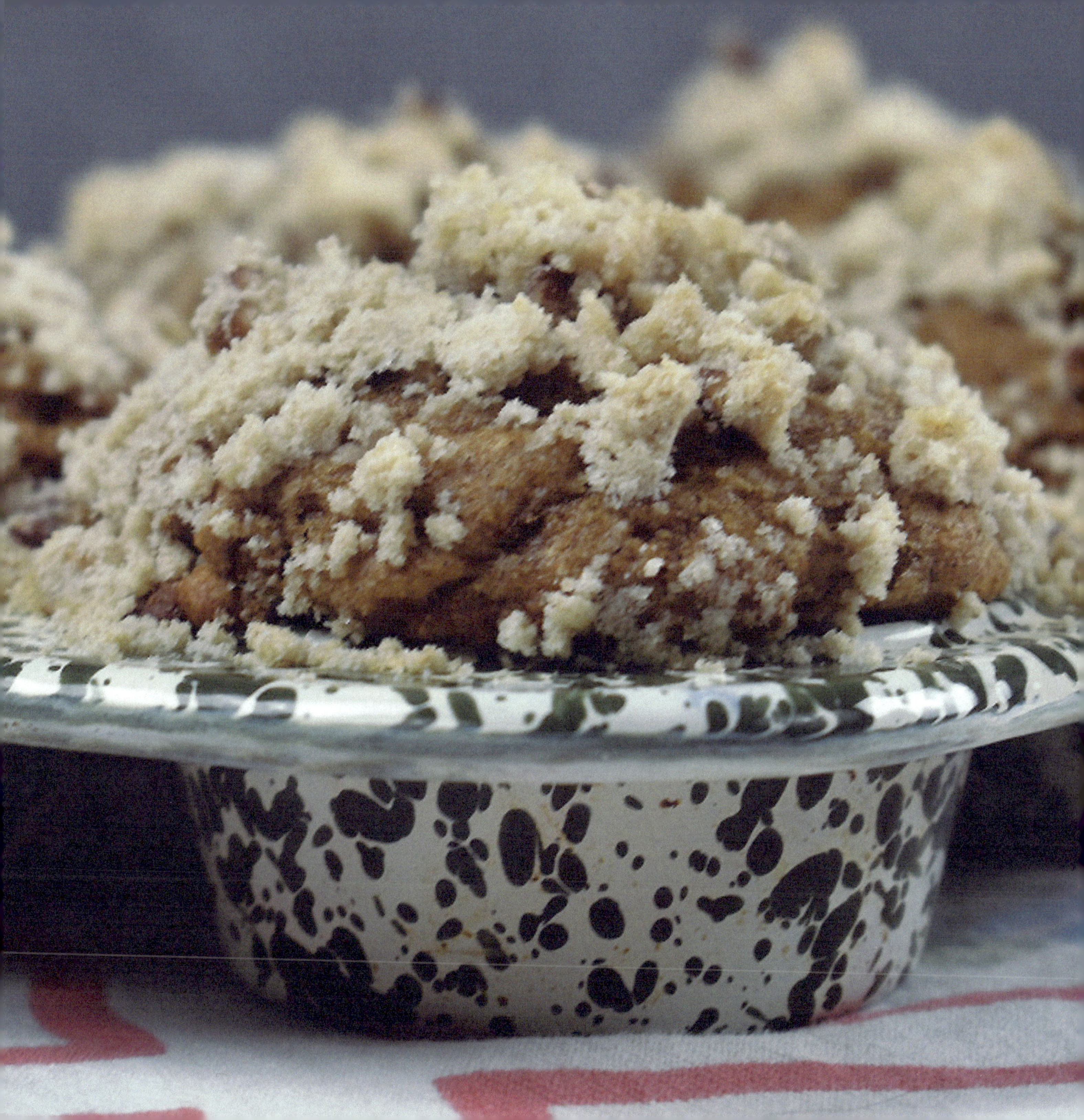

Apple Butter Spice Muffins

1 ½ cups white whole wheat flour
½ cup white flour
2 teaspoons baking powder
⅛ teaspoon salt
1 teaspoon cinnamon
¼ teaspoon nutmeg
⅛ teaspoon allspice
½ cup honey
2 Tablespoons oil
⅓ cup apple butter
1 cup milk
1 egg
Topping: ½ cup chopped walnuts or pecans, and cinnamon sugar.

A richer, spicier version of applesauce muffins, yet just as easy to fix.

1. Preheat oven to 350 degrees F.
2. Mix together the dry ingredients.
3. Add wet ingredients, stirring just to combine (avoid overmixing).
4. Spoon batter into muffin cups, and sprinkle with nuts and cinnamon sugar.
5. Bake for 15-18 minutes. (Best not to overbake) Makes 12 muffins.

Per Muffin

Calories: 185
Fat: 6g
Cholesterol: 15mg
Sodium: 112mg

Potassium: 14mg
Carbs: 29g
Fiber: 2g
Sugars: 15g
Protein: 4g

Vitamin A: 1%
Vitamin C: 0%
Calcium: 49%
Iron: 5%

Moist Applesauce Bran Muffins

Full of wholesomeness, with every ingredient.

- 1 cup unprocessed wheat bran
- 1 ½ cups whole wheat flour
- ⅛ teaspoon salt
- ½ cup raisins
- 1 teaspoon baking powder
- 1 teaspoon baking soda
- 1 cup milk
- ¼ cup honey
- ¼ cup molasses
- ¾ cup applesauce
- 2 Tablespoons oil
- 2 eggs
- 1 teaspoon vanilla
- Topping: ⅓ cup pecans

1. Preheat oven to 350 degrees F.
2. Mix together the dry ingredients.
3. Stir the raisins into the dry ingredients.
4. Make a well in the center and add the wet ingredients, stirring just to combine. The batter will seem a bit runny – not to worry.
5. Spoon batter into muffin cups. Sprinkle with pecans.
6. Bake 15-18 minutes. Makes 12 muffins. (Pour any extra batter into a mini bundt pan for a darling little cake.)

Per Muffin

Calories: 185
Fat: 5g
Cholesterol: 31mg
Sodium: 156mg

Potassium: 192mg
Carbs: 33g
Fiber: 5g
Sugars: 16g
Protein: 5g

Vitamin A: 1%
Vitamin C: 13%
Calcium: 26%
Iron: 8%

Apple Crumble Muffins

½ cup whole wheat flour
½ cup white whole wheat flour
1 cup white flour
⅛ teaspoon salt
1 teaspoon baking soda
3 Tablespoons brown sugar
2 teaspoons apple pie spice
1 egg
1 apple, peeled and grated
½ cup buttermilk
1 teaspoon vanilla
½ cup honey
2 Tablespoons oil
½ cup raisins

Crumble Topping:
⅓ cup white flour
3 Tablespoons sugar
1 Tablespoon butter
¼ teaspoon cinnamon
¼ cup pecans, chopped

One bite and you'll wonder where these muffins have been all your life.

1. Preheat oven to 350 degrees.
2. In a small bowl, prepare the Crumble Topping by blending together flour, sugar and cinnamon. Rub in the butter until crumbly. Stir in the pecans. Set aside.
3. While preparing the muffins, soak the raisins in boiling water to plump them up a bit.
4. Blend together the wet ingredients in a medium size bowl.
5. Add the grated apple. Drain the raisins.
6. In a separate bowl, blend the dry ingredients and then combine with the wet ingredients, along with the drained raisins.
7. Spoon batter into muffin cups and, using your fingers, top with the crumble topping.
8. Bake for 16-18 minutes. (Best not to overbake). Makes 12 muffins.

Per Muffin

Calories: 185
Fat: 3g
Cholesterol: 16mg
Sodium: 116mg
Potassium: 81mg
Carbs: 37g
Fiber: 2g
Sugars: 20g
Protein: 4g
Vitamin A: 1%
Vitamin C: 1%
Calcium: 3%
Iron: 3%

Per Crumb Topping

Calories: 45
Fat: 2g
Cholesterol: 3mg
Sodium: 0mg
Potassium: 1mg
Carbs: 6g
Fiber: 0g
Sugars: 3g
Protein: 1g
Vitamin A: 8%
Vitamin C: 0%
Calcium: 0%
Iron: 0%

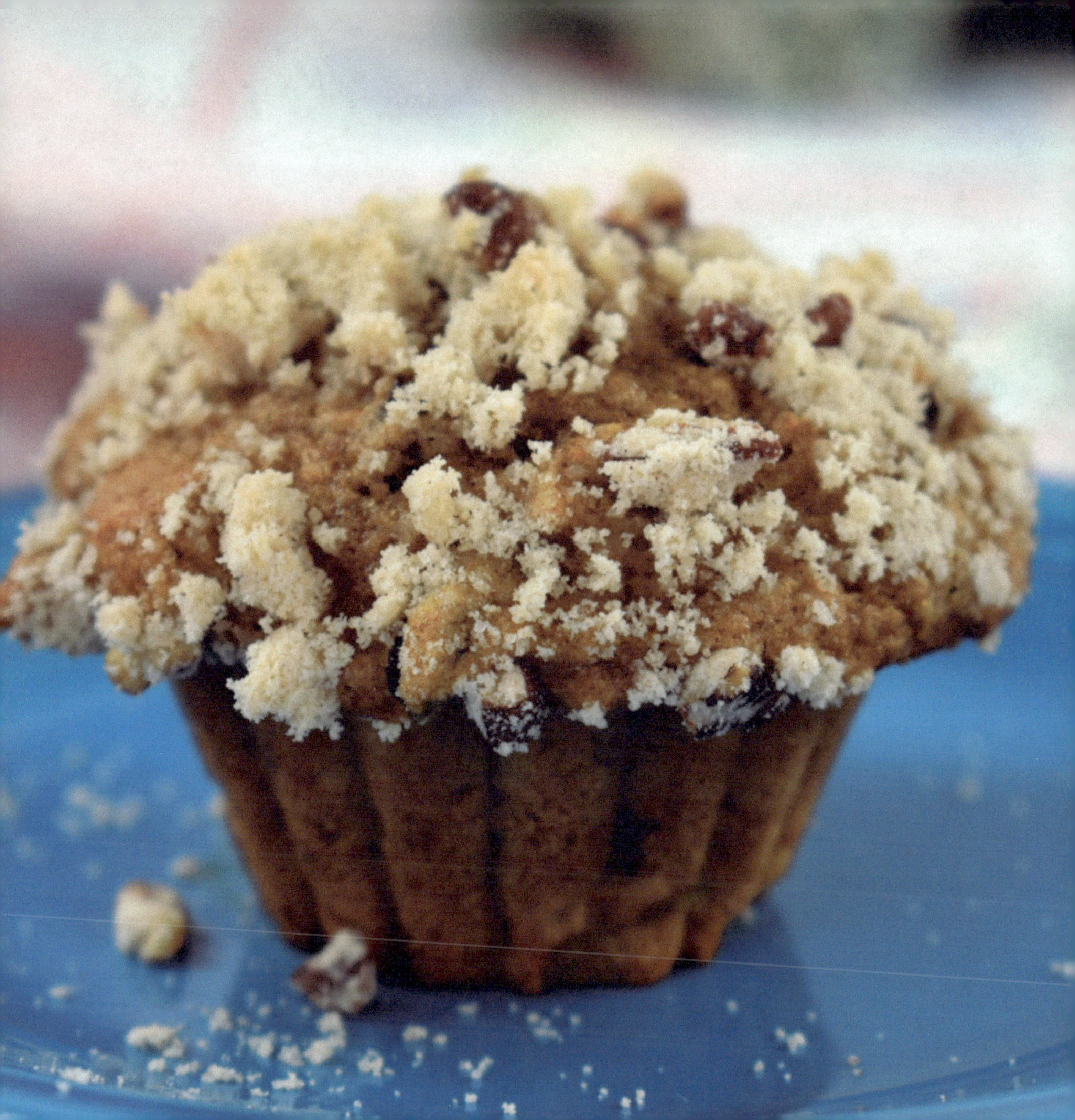

Applesauce Spice Muffins

¾ cup whole wheat flour
¾ cup white whole wheat flour
½ cup white flour
1 Tablespoon baking powder
⅛ teaspoon salt
1 ¼ teaspoons cinnamon
¼ teaspoon nutmeg
Pinch cloves
½ cup honey
1 cup applesauce
1 teaspoon vanilla
2 Tablespoons oil
½ cup milk
1 egg
Topping: Cinnamon sugar

A simple, quick, and satisfying muffin any day of the week.

1. Preheat oven to 350 degrees F.
2. Mix together the dry ingredients.
3. Make a well in the center and add wet ingredients, stirring just to combine (avoid overmixing).
4. Spoon batter into muffin cups. Sprinkle with cinnamon sugar.
5. Bake for 15-18 minutes. (Best if a bit underbaked.) Makes 12 muffins.

Per Muffin

Calories: 135
Fat: 3g
Cholesterol: 16mg
Sodium: 157mg
Potassium: 58mg
Carbs: 25g
Fiber: 1g
Sugars: 16g
Protein: 3g
Vitamin A: 3%
Vitamin C: 1%
Calcium: 82%
Iron: 3%

Sunny Apricot Muffins

Sweet and floral, a great muffin to usher in spring.

1 cup white flour
1 cup white whole wheat flour
1 Tablespoon baking powder
⅛ teaspoon salt
½ teaspoon cardamom
½ cup honey
2 Tablespoons brown sugar
1 egg
½ teaspoon vanilla
A drop of almond extract
2 Tablespoons oil
1 Can (14 oz.) apricot halves, packed in fruit juice*
⅓ cup buttermilk
Topping: ½ cup slivered almonds and sugar for sprinkling.

1. Preheat oven to 350 degrees F.
2. Drain the apricots and purée them in a blender. (This will yield about 1 cup pureed fruit.)
3. Mix the dry ingredients together.
4. Add wet ingredients, including the puréed apricots.
5. Spoon batter into muffin cups. Sprinkle with nuts and sugar.
6. Bake for 15-18 minutes. (Best if a bit underbaked.) Makes 12 muffins.
7. Note: canned peaches also work nicely

Per Muffin

Calories: 201
Fat: 5g
Cholesterol: 16mg
Sodium: 165mg

Potassium: 96mg
Carbs: 34g
Fiber: 2g
Sugars: 18g
Protein: 4g

Vitamin A: 17%
Vitamin C: 1%
Calcium: 76%
Iron: 4%

Chapter 7
Dried Fruit for Dolce Vita

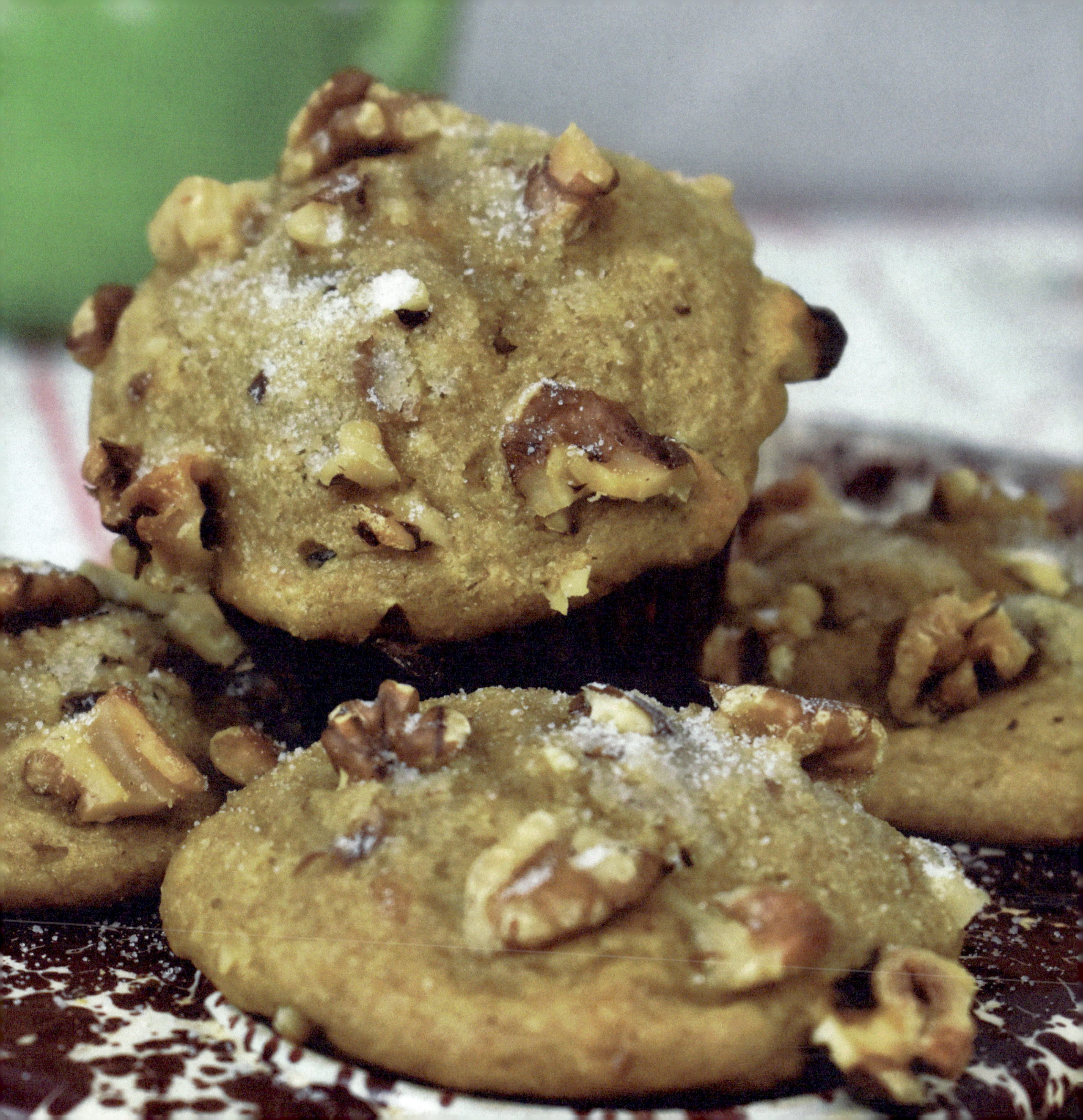

Apricot Streusel Muffins

1 cup white whole wheat flour
1 cup white flour
½ cup honey
¾ cup dried apricots, chopped
1 teaspoon baking powder
½ teaspoon baking soda
⅛ teaspoon salt
1 cup buttermilk
¼ cup butter, melted
1 egg
1 teaspoon vanilla
¼ teaspoon almond extract

Streusel Topping:
2 Tablespoons flour
2 Tablespoons sugar
1 teaspoon cinnamon
2 teaspoons butter
½ cup slivered almonds

A delicate muffin for the almond lover.

1. Preheat oven to 350 degrees F.
2. In a small bowl, mix together the crumble topping by first blending the flour, sugar, and cinnamon. Rub in the butter until crumbly. Stir in the almonds. Set aside.
3. Combine the dry ingredients for the muffin.
4. Rub the dried apricots into the dry ingredients to prevent clumping.
5. Add the wet ingredients, stirring just to combine (best not to overmix). Spoon batter into muffin cups.
6. Sprinkle with streusel topping.
7. Bake 15-18 minutes. (Best when a bit underbaked.) Makes 12 muffins.

Per Muffin

Calories: 169
Fat: 5g
Cholesterol: 26mg
Sodium: 130mg
Potassium: 1mg
Carbs: 28g
Fiber: 1g
Sugars: 13g
Protein: 4g
Vitamin A: 33%
Vitamin C: 1%
Calcium: 28%
Iron: 3%

Per Streusel

Calories: 61
Fat: 5g
Cholesterol: 5mg
Sodium: 47mg
Potassium: 2mg
Carbs: 3g
Fiber: 0g
Sugars: 2g
Protein: 1g
Vitamin A: 16%
Vitamin C: 0%
Calcium: 3%
Iron: 0%

Apple Oat Bran Muffins

Moist and flavorful, these will keep you going all morning.

1 ½ Sweet apples
1 egg
½ cup plus apple cider (or juice)
3 Tablespoons oil
1/3 cup honey
2 Tablespoons brown sugar
1 cup oat bran
½ cup white whole wheat flour
½ cup white flour
2 teaspoons baking powder
¼ teaspoon salt
1 teaspoon cinnamon
½ teaspoon vanilla-orange extract
½ cup raisins
Topping: Cinnamon Sugar

1. Preheat oven to 350 degrees F.
2. In a small bowl, soak the raisins in hot water while you prepare the muffins.
3. Grate the apple, unpeeled, using the largest side of a cheese grater.
4. In a medium bowl, combine the oat bran, grated apple, apple juice, egg, oil, honey, and vanilla-orange extract. Let stand for 5 minutes.
5. In a large bowl, mix together the remaining dry ingredients. Drain the raisins.
6. Make a well in the center, and add wet ingredients, including raisins, stirring just to combine.
7. Spoon batter into muffin cups. Sprinkle with cinnamon sugar.
8. Bake for 15-18 minutes. (Best if a bit underbaked.) Makes 12 muffins.

Per Muffin

Calories: 190
Fat: 4g
Cholesterol: 16mg
Sodium: 144mg

Potassium: 45mg
Carbs: 35g
Fiber: 4g
Sugars: 18g
Protein: 4g

Vitamin A: 7%
Vitamin C: 2%
Calcium: 9%
Iron: 5%

Date Nut Muffins

- ¾ cup whole wheat flour
- ¾ cup white whole wheat flour
- ½ cup white flour
- ⅛ teaspoon salt
- ½ cup honey
- ½ teaspoon baking soda
- ½ cup low-fat sour cream
- 2 eggs
- 1 teaspoon vanilla
- ½ cup applesauce
- 2 Tablespoons oil
- 2 Tablespoons milk
- ½ cup chopped dates
- Topping: ½ cup chopped walnuts and white sugar for sprinkling

Reliably moist and satisfying.

1. Preheat oven to 350 degrees F.
2. In a medium bowl, mix together dry ingredients.
3. Stir the chopped dates into the dry ingredients (to prevent clumping).
4. Make a well in the center and add the wet ingredients.
5. Stir just to combine (avoid overmixing).
6. Spoon batter into muffin cups and sprinkle walnuts over top, followed by a sprinkling of white sugar.
7. Bake for 15-18 minutes. (Best if a bit underbaked.) Makes 12 muffins.

Per Muffin

Calories: 229
Fat: 7g
Cholesterol: 36mg
Sodium: 86mg

Potassium: 105mg
Carbs: 37g
Fiber: 3g
Sugars: 23g
Protein: 5g

Vitamin A: 15%
Vitamin C: 8%
Calcium: 14%
Iron: 3%

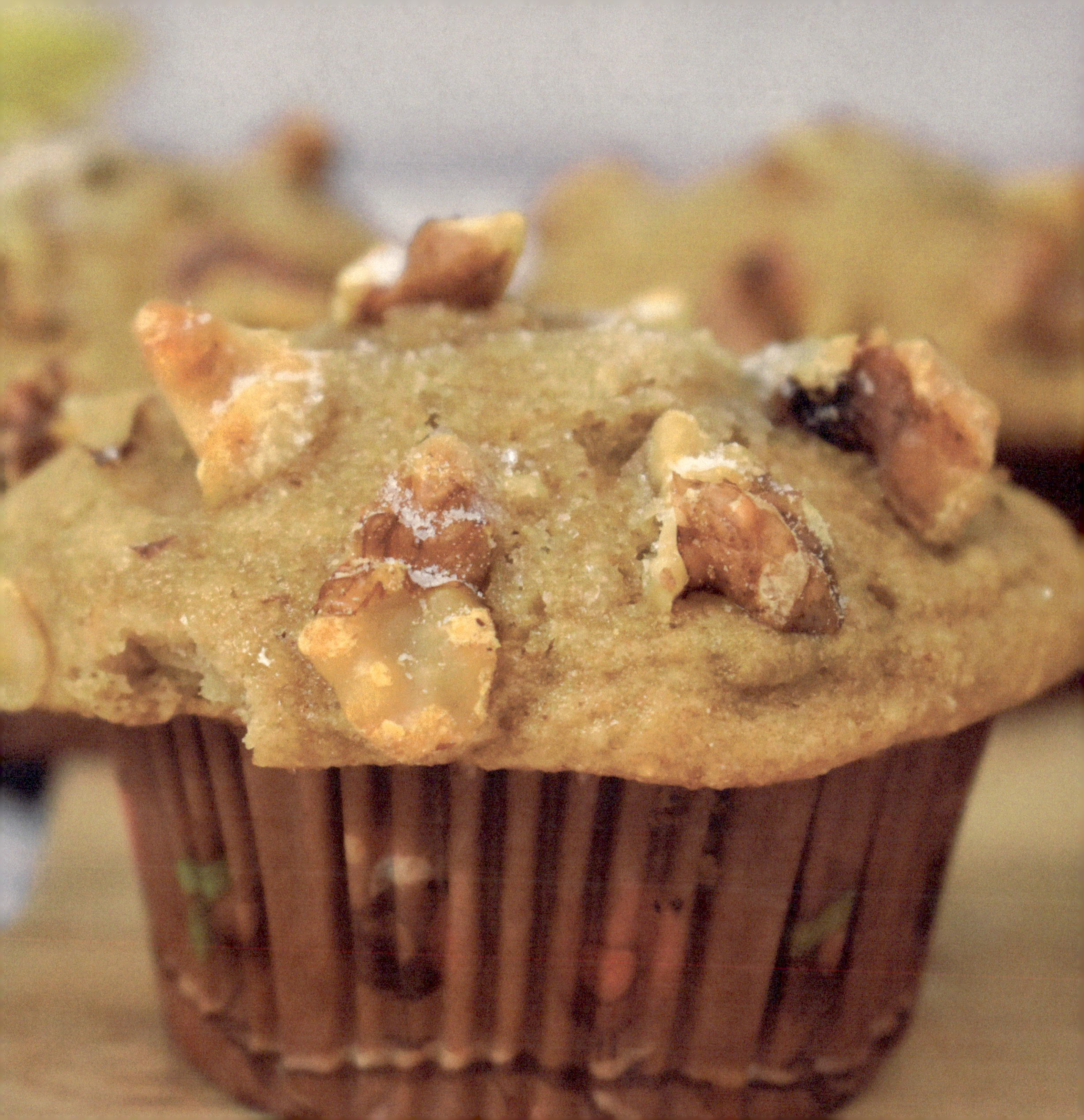

Lemon Apricot Muffins

½ cup whole wheat flour
½ cup white whole wheat flour
1 cup white flour
½ teaspoon baking soda
⅛ teaspoon salt
½ cup honey
½ cup low-fat sour cream
½ teaspoon vanilla
Grated rind of one lemon
2 Tablespoons oil
2 Tablespoons milk
2 eggs
¾ cup chopped dried apricots
Topping: Sugar for sprinkling

A summery muffin for the screened-in porch.

1. Preheat oven to 350 degrees F.
2. While mixing dry ingredients, soak the chopped dried apricots in boiling water.
3. Drain the apricots completely.
4. Add the wet ingredients to dry ingredients, along with the apricots, then the lemon rind, stirring just to combine.
5. Spoon batter into muffin cups, sprinkle with sugar.
6. Bake for 15-18 minutes. (Best if slightly underbaked.) Makes 12 muffins.

Per Muffin

Calories: 186
Fat: 4g
Cholesterol: 34mg
Sodium: 85mg
Potassium: 124mg
Carbs: 33g
Fiber: 2g
Sugars: 18g
Protein: 5g
Vitamin A: 10%
Vitamin C: 1%
Calcium: 4%
Iron: 4%

Cherry Danish Muffins

Special yet surprisingly simple.

1 ½ cups white whole wheat flour
½ cup white flour
1 Tablespoon baking powder
⅛ teaspoon salt
½ cup chopped dried cherries
¼ cup white chocolate chips
¾ cup buttermilk
2 Tablespoons apple juice
1 egg
½ cup honey
½ teaspoon vanilla
¼ teaspoon almond extract
3 Tablespoons oil
Topping: Sugar and ½ cup slivered almonds for sprinkling.

1. Preheat oven to 350 degrees F.
2. Mix together the dry ingredients.
3. Add wet ingredients, along with chopped cherries and white chocolate chips, stirring just to combine.
4. Spoon batter into muffin cups.
5. Sprinkle with almonds followed by sugar.
6. Bake 15-18 minutes. (Always best not to overbake.) Makes 12 muffins.

Per Muffin

Calories: 240
Fat: 9g
Cholesterol: 16mg
Sodium: 174mg

Potassium: 83mg
Carbs: 37g
Fiber: 3g
Sugars: 20g
Protein: 5g

Vitamin A: 6%
Vitamin C: 2%
Calcium: 88%
Iron: 2%

Oatmeal Date Muffins

¾ cup whole wheat flour
½ cup white flour
1 cup rolled oats
⅛ teaspoon salt
1 Tablespoon baking powder
¼ teaspoon salt
½ cup honey
½ cup chopped dates
1 egg
⅓ cup applesauce
2 Tablespoons oil
1 cup milk
Topping: Chopped walnuts (optional).

A straightforward muffin to fortify you.

1. Preheat oven to 350 degrees F.
2. In a medium bowl, mix together the dry ingredients.
3. Add chopped dates into dry ingredients and rub into the flour mixture (this will prevent clumping).
4. Make a well in the center and add wet ingredients.
5. Stir just to combine (avoid overmixing).
6. Spoon batter into muffin cups.
7. Bake for 15-18 minutes. (Best if not overbaked.) Makes 12 muffins.

Per Muffin

Calories: 190
Fat: 4g
Cholesterol: 17mg
Sodium: 212mg

Potassium: 122mg
Carbs: 37g
Fiber: 3g
Sugars: 21g
Protein: 4g

Vitamin A: 6%
Vitamin C: 6%
Calcium: 94%
Iron: 3%

Fig Hazelnut Muffins

Full of intense, warm wholesomeness.

1 cup white flour
1 cup whole wheat flour
2 Tablespoons wheat germ
⅛ teaspoon salt
½ cup honey
1 teaspoon baking soda
1 teaspoon cinnamon
1 teaspoon ginger
¼ teaspoon allspice
a pinch of nutmeg
½ cup applesauce
⅓ cup molasses
⅔ cup buttermilk
2 eggs
2 Tablespoons oil
10 figs, chopped (I use Mission figs)
Topping: ½ cup chopped hazelnuts, and cinnamon sugar for sprinkling.

1. Preheat oven to 350 degrees F.
2. In a medium bowl, mix together dry ingredients.
3. Stir the chopped figs into dry ingredients (this will prevent clumping).
4. Make a well in the center and add the wet ingredients.
5. Stir just to combine (avoid overmixing).
6. Spoon batter into muffin cups. Sprinkle hazelnuts on top, followed by cinnamon sugar.
7. Bake for 15-18 minutes. (Best if a bit underbaked.) Makes 12 muffins.

Per Muffin

Calories: 248
Fat: 6g
Cholesterol: 32mg
Sodium: 131mg

Potassium: 38mg
Carbs: 42g
Fiber: 3g
Sugars: 23g
Protein: 6g

Vitamin A: 15%
Vitamin C: 9%
Calcium: 14%
Iron: 6%

Chapter 8
Spices for Serenity

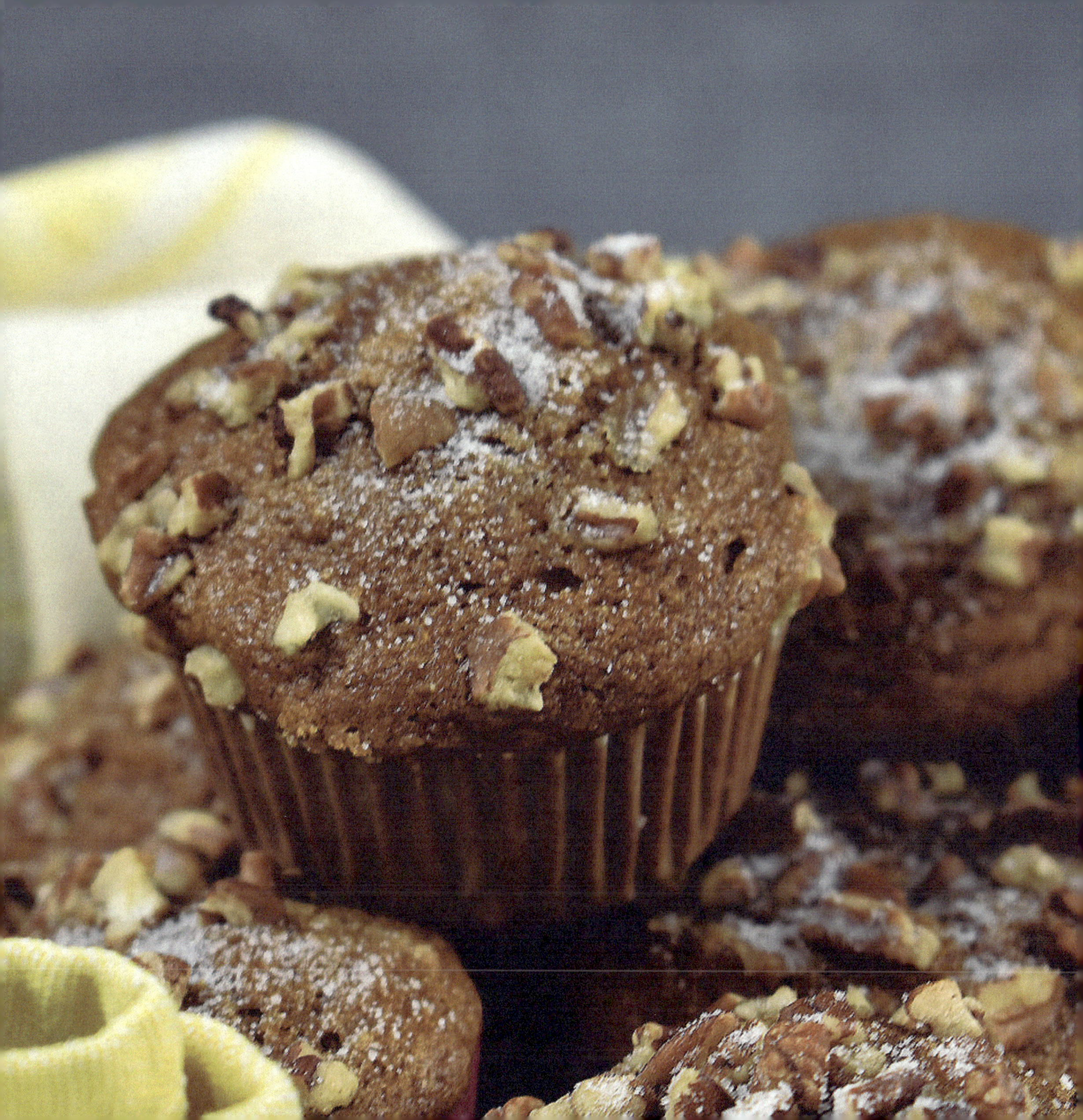

Rum-Raisin Spice Muffins

- 1 cup white flour
- ⅔ cup white whole wheat flour
- ⅓ cup wheat bran
- 1 ¼ teaspoons baking powder
- 1 teaspoons cinnamon
- ¾ teaspoon baking soda
- ⅛ teaspoon salt
- ¾ cup raisins
- 3 Tablespoons rum
- ½ cup honey
- 1 cup buttermilk
- 3 Tablespoons oil
- 1 egg
- 1 ½ teaspoons vanilla

Topping: Sugar for sprinkling.

Something a bit more exotic to start the day.

1. Preheat oven to 350 degrees F.
2. In a small bowl, soak the raisins in boiling water.
3. Meanwhile, combine the dry ingredients.
4. Drain the raisins completely.
5. Add wet ingredients, along with soaked raisins, stirring just to combine.
6. Spoon batter into muffin cups.
7. Sprinkle with sugar.
8. Bake 15-18 minutes. (Always best slightly underbaked.) Makes 12 muffins.

Per Muffin

Calories: 189
Fat: 4g
Cholesterol: 16mg
Sodium: 110mg

Potassium: 181mg
Carbs: 34g
Fiber: 2g
Sugars: 19g
Protein: 4g

Vitamin A: 1%
Vitamin C: 0%
Calcium: 7%
Iron: 4%

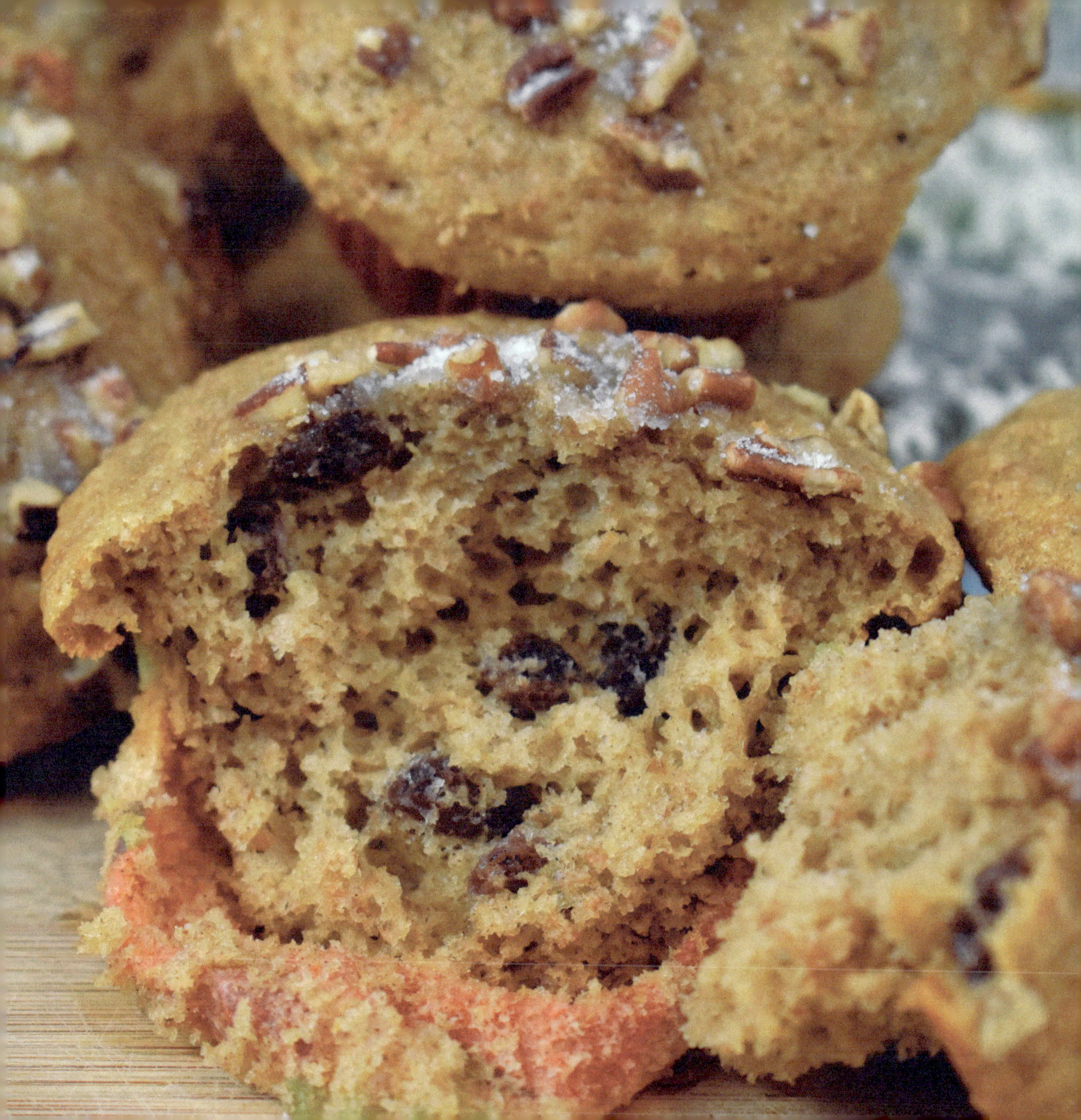

Anise Muffins

½ cup whole wheat flour
½ cup white whole wheat flour
1 cup white flour
⅛ teaspoon salt
½ cup honey
½ teaspoon baking soda
1 teaspoon ground anise
2 Tablespoons oil
½ cup applesauce
½ cup low-fat sour cream
1 teaspoon vanilla
2 eggs
2 Tablespoons milk
½ cup raisins
Topping: ½ cup chopped almonds, and sugar for sprinkling.

A cozy muffin indeed, with an underrated spice.

1. Preheat oven to 350 degrees F.
2. In a small bowl, soak the raisins in some boiling water while you measure and mix the dry ingredients.
3. Mix the dry ingredients together in a medium bowl. Add the wet ingredients.
4. Drain the raisins and add them to the mixture.
5. Mix until just blended (avoid overmixing).
6. Spoon batter into muffin cups. Sprinkle almonds over top, followed by sugar.
7. Bake for 16-18 minutes. (Best if a bit underbaked.) Makes 12 muffins.

Per Muffin

Calories: 209
Fat: 6g
Cholesterol: 36mg
Sodium: 125mg

Potassium: 75mg
Carbs: 34g
Fiber: 2g
Sugars: 17g
Protein: 5g

Vitamin A: 15%
Vitamin C: 8%
Calcium: 19%
Iron: 3%

Cinnamony Muffins

(an eggless muffin)

Great if you need an eggless muffin, but don't let that stop you from making these super moist, healthful muffins any time.

1 cup whole wheat flour
1 cup white flour
¾ teaspoon cinnamon
pinch cloves
⅛ teaspoon salt
1 cup applesauce
1 ½ teaspoons baking powder
½ teaspoon baking soda
¼ cup honey
¼ cup molasses
2 Tablespoons oil
½ cup raisins
Topping: ⅓ cup Pecans

1. Preheat oven to 350 degrees F.
2. In a small bowl, soak the raisins in boiling water for a few minutes.
3. In a medium bowl, mix together the dry ingredients.
4. Drain the raisins thoroughly.
5. Make a well in the center and add wet ingredients, along with the raisins.
6. Stir just to combine (avoid overmixing).
7. Spoon batter into muffin cups. Sprinkle with pecans.
8. Bake for 15-18 minutes. (Always best not to overbake.) Makes 12 muffins.

Per Muffin

Calories: 176
Fat: 4g
Cholesterol: 0mg
Sodium: 128mg

Potassium: 182mg
Carbs: 33g
Fiber: 2g
Sugars: 17g
Protein: 3g

Vitamin A: 0%
Vitamin C: 17%
Calcium: 38%
Iron: 4%

Glazed Chai Latte Muffins

½ cup whole wheat flour
½ cup white whole wheat flour
1 cup white flour
1 teaspoon baking powder
½ teaspoon baking soda
⅛ teaspoon salt
1 Tablespoon Chai spice mix (see below)
2 Tablespoons oil
½ cup honey with a bit of molasses
¾-1 cup buttermilk
1 egg
2 teaspoons vanilla
½ cup chopped dates

Chai Spice Mix
1 teaspoon cardamon
1 teaspoon ginger
1 teaspoon cinnamon
½ teaspoon allspice
¼ teaspoon white pepper

Glaze
¼ cup powdered sugar
3 oz. cream cheese
¼ teaspoon vanilla
some milk

A bit more involved and rich, but great for a special morning, or to make the morning special.

1. Preheat oven to 350 degrees F.
2. Mix together the dry ingredients.
3. Rub the dates into the dry ingredients to prevent clumping.
4. As you measure the honey, just before you reach the top of the measure, top it off with molasses (2-3 tablespoons worth).
5. Combine the wet and dry ingredients, stirring just to combine, with enough buttermilk to create a thick batter.
6. Spoon batter into muffin cups. Bake 15-18 minutes. (Important not to overbake these). Makes 12 muffins.
7. Mix the glaze ingredients and cover to prevent hardening.
8. After muffins are done baking, spread glaze over the warm muffins.

Per Muffin

Calories: 185
Fat: 3g
Cholesterol: 16mg
Sodium: 130mg
Potassium: 128mg
Carbs: 36g
Fiber: 2g
Sugars: 21g
Protein: 4g
Vitamin A: 1%
Vitamin C: 0%
Calcium: 27%
Iron: 3%

Per Glaze

Calories: 23
Fat: 1g
Cholesterol: 4mg
Sodium: 22mg
Potassium: 0mg
Carbs: 3g
Fiber: 0g
Sugars: 3g
Protein: 1g
Vitamin A: 1%
Vitamin C: 0%
Calcium: 0%
Iron: 0%

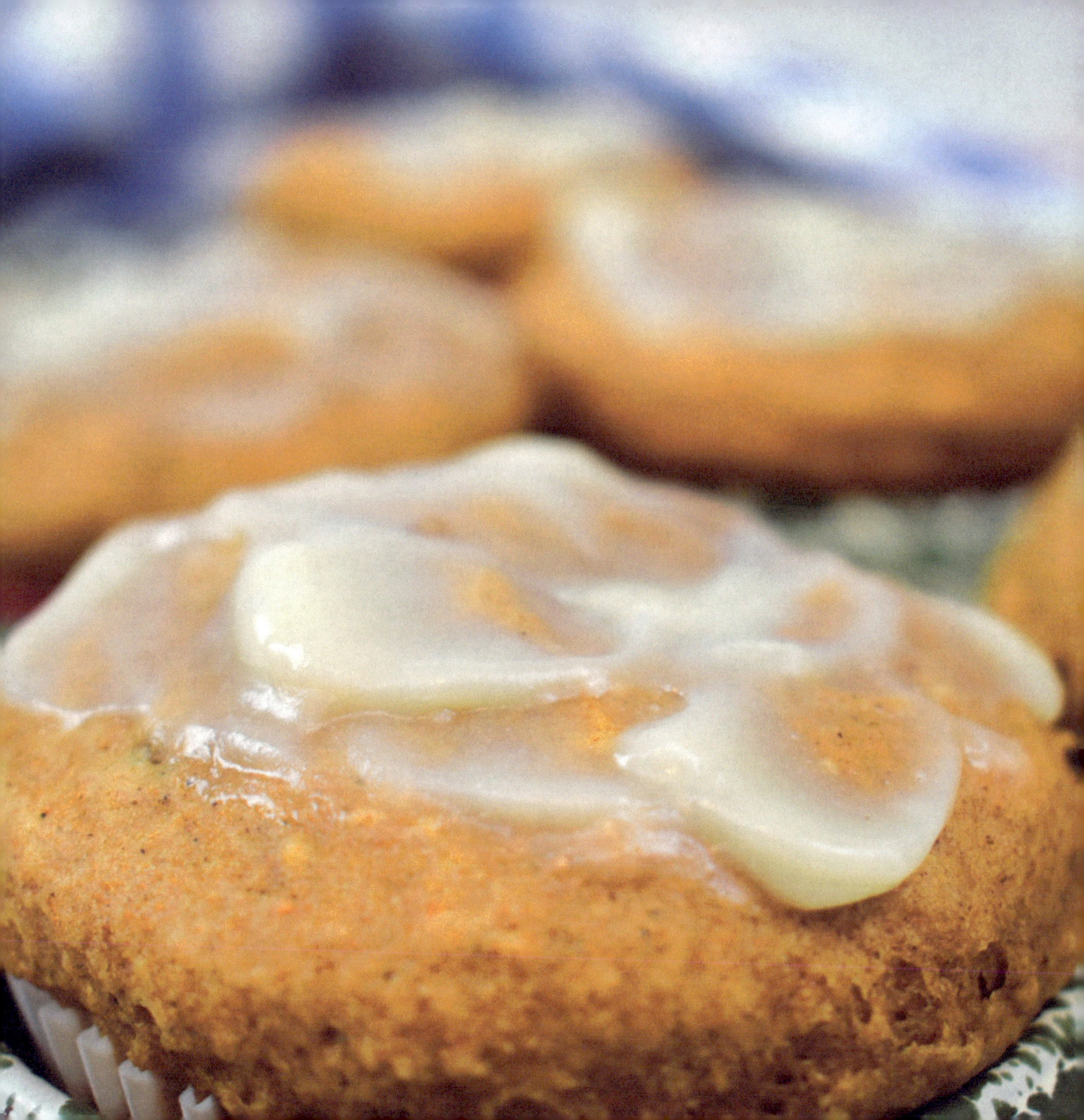

Fresh Ginger Muffins

- 1 cup white whole wheat flour
- 1 cup white flour
- ⅛ teaspoon salt
- ½ cup honey
- ½ teaspoon baking soda
- 2 Tablespoons grated fresh ginger root
- 2 Tablespoons oil
- ½ cup applesauce
- ½ cup low-fat sour cream
- 1 teaspoon vanilla
- 2 eggs
- 2 Tablespoons milk
- Topping: 3 Tablespoons sesame seeds and sugar for sprinkling

The fresh ginger in these makes for an especially nice pick-me-up.

1. Preheat oven to 350 degrees F.
2. Mix dry ingredients together in a medium bowl.
3. Add the wet ingredients, and mix until just blended (avoid overmixing).
4. Spoon batter into muffin cups, and sprinkle with sesame seeds followed by sugar.
5. Bake for 16-18 minutes. (Best if a bit underbaked.) Makes 12 muffins.

Per Muffin

Calories: 172
Fat: 5g
Cholesterol: 36mg
Sodium: 87mg
Potassium: 48mg
Carbs: 29g
Fiber: 1g
Sugars: 14g
Protein: 4g
Vitamin A: 15%
Vitamin C: 9%
Calcium: 9%
Iron: 3%

Coffee Cinnamon Muffins

Think your favorite coffee shop on a cozy afternoon

½ cup whole wheat flour
½ cup white whole wheat flour
1 cup white flour
⅛ teaspoon salt
½ teaspoon baking soda
⅔ cup honey
1 ½ teaspoons cinnamon
¼ cup powdered coffee dissolved in
2 Tablespoons of water
⅔ cup applesauce
1 egg
½ cup buttermilk
1 teaspoon vanilla
2 Tablespoons oil
Topping: Cinnamon sugar for sprinkling

1. Preheat oven to 350 degrees F.
2. In a medium bowl, mix together the dry ingredients.
3. Make a well in the center and add wet ingredients.
4. Stir just to combine (avoid overmixing).
5. Spoon batter into muffin cups and sprinkle with cinnamon sugar.
6. Bake for 16 minutes. (Best if a bit underbaked.) Makes 12 muffins.

Per Muffin

Calories: 170
Fat: 3g
Cholesterol: 16mg
Sodium: 87mg

Potassium: 71mg
Carbs: 32g
Fiber: 1g
Sugars: 17g
Protein: 3g

Vitamin A: 0%
Vitamin C: 11%
Calcium: 7%
Iron: 2%

Gingerbread Muffins

- ½ cup whole wheat flour
- ½ cup white whole wheat flour
- ¾ cup white flour
- ⅛ teaspoon salt
- 1 teaspoon baking soda
- 2 teaspoons ground ginger
- 1 teaspoon cinnamon
- ⅛ teaspoon cloves
- ⅛ teaspoon nutmeg
- ½ cup applesauce
- ¼ cup honey
- ¼ cup molasses
- ⅔ cup buttermilk
- 2 eggs
- 2 Tablespoons oil
- ½ cup raisins
- Topping: sugar for sprinkling

A kid favorite, and a heart-warming surprise for a friend or neighbor.

1. Preheat oven to 350 degrees F.
2. In a small bowl, soak the raisins in boiling water for a few minutes to plump them up.
3. Mix the dry ingredients together.
4. Drain the raisins thoroughly.
5. Mix in the wet ingredients, along with the raisins, and stir until just blended (avoid overmixing).
6. Spoon the batter into the muffin pan. Sprinkle with sugar.
7. Bake for 15-18 minutes (with these, it's super important not to over-bake). Makes 12 muffins.

Per Muffin

Calories: 167	**Potassium:** 91mg	**Vitamin A:** 14%
Fat: 3g	**Carbs:** 30g	**Vitamin C:** 9%
Cholesterol: 32mg	**Fiber:** 2g	**Calcium:** 11%
Sodium: 133mg	**Sugars:** 14g	**Iron:** 5%

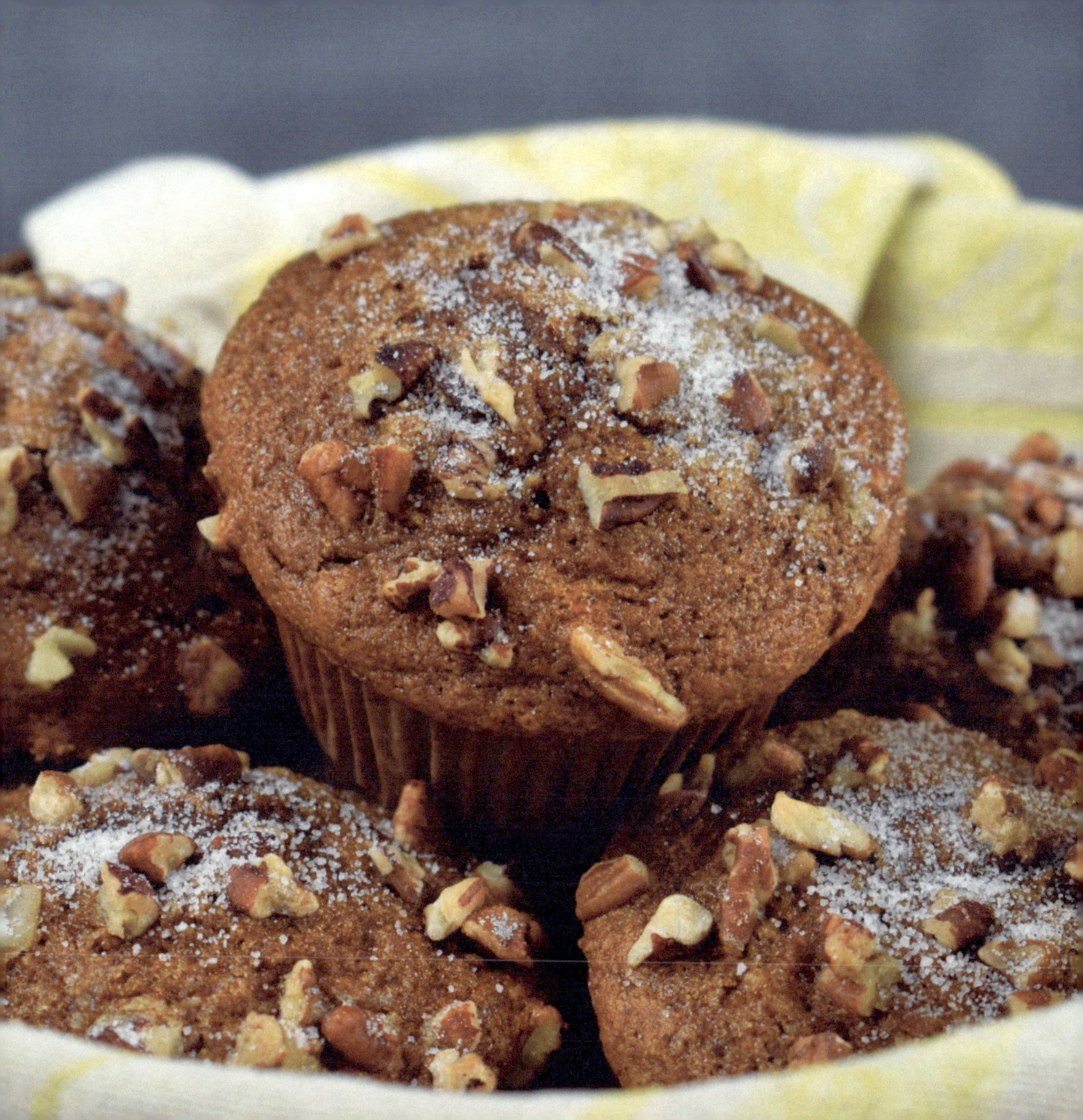

Christmas Morning Muffins

1 ½ cups white whole wheat flour
½ cup white flour
1 Tablespoon baking powder
⅛ teaspoon salt
2 Tablespoons sugar
½ teaspoon cinnamon
½ cup honey
2 eggs
½ cup applesauce
2 Tablespoons oil
1 teaspoon vanilla
2-3 Tablespoons rum
⅓ cup milk
¼ cup dried cranberries, finely chopped
⅓ cup raisins
Topping: ⅓ cup pecans and sugar

The flavors of the festive season in a muffin. I only make these at holiday time, which makes them even more special.

1. Preheat oven to 350 degrees F.
2. In a small bowl, soak the raisins in boiling water for a few minutes to plump them up, and to prevent them from drying out the muffin.
3. Meanwhile, mix together the dry ingredients.
4. Rub the dried cranberries into dry ingredients (to prevent clumping later).
5. Drain the raisins thoroughly.
6. Add wet ingredients, along with the raisins, stirring just to combine.
7. Spoon batter into muffin cups, and sprinkle with pecans and sugar.
8. Bake for 15-18 minutes. (Best when slightly underbaked). Makes 12 muffins.

Per Muffin

Calories: 191
Fat: 4g
Cholesterol: 31mg
Sodium: 161mg
Potassium: 62mg
Carbs: 33g
Fiber: 2g
Sugars: 18g
Protein: 4g
Vitamin A: 1%
Vitamin C: 9%
Calcium: 71%
Iron: 5%

Index

Index

Index

Index

Made in the USA
Las Vegas, NV
02 November 2026

57098958R10061